a LANGE medical book

CURRENT
Practice Guidelines
in Inpatient Medicine
2018–2019

Jacob A. David, MD, FAAFP
Associate Program Director
Ventura County Medical Center Family Medicine Residency Program
Clinical Instructor, Family Medicine, UCLA David Geffen School of Medicine
Ventura, California

New York   Chicago   San Francisco   Athens   London   Madrid
Mexico City   Milan   New Delhi   Singapore   Sydney   Toronto

CURRENT Practice Guidelines in Inpatient Medicine, 2018–2019

1 2 3 4 5 6 7 8 9   LCR   23 22 21 20 19 18

ISBN 978-1-260-01222-4
MHID 1-260-01222-0

This book was set in Minion Pro by MPS Limited.
The editors were Amanda Fielding and Kim J. Davis.
The production supervisor was Catherine Saggese.
Project management was provided by Vivek Khandelwal, MPS Limited.

This book is printed on acid-free paper.

Library of Congress Cataloging-in-Publication Data

Names: David, Jacob A., author.
Title: Current practice guidelines in inpatient medicine 2018-2019 / Jacob A. David, MD, FAAFP, Associate Program Director, Ventura County Medical Center Family Medicine Residency Program, Clinical Instructor, UCLA David Geffen School of Medicine, Ventura, California.
Description: New York : McGraw-Hill Education, [2018] | Includes bibliographical references and index. |
Identifiers: LCCN 2017059443 (print) | LCCN 2018004019 (ebook) | ISBN 9781260012231 (ebook) | ISBN 1260012239 (ebook) | ISBN 9781260012224 (paperback) | ISBN 1260012220 (paperback)
Subjects: LCSH: Internal medicine. | Medicine—Practice. | BISAC: MEDICAL /Internal Medicine.
Classification: LCC RC46 (ebook) | LCC RC46 .D235 2018 (print) | DDC 616.0068—dc23
LC record available at https://lccn.loc.gov/2017059443

This book is dedicated to the VCMC Family Medicine family, and to Ken and Karen, who helped with homework.

Contents

6. INFECTIOUS DISEASE
Neil Jorgensen and Marina Morie

7. HEMATOLOGY
Tipu V. Khan, Seth Alkire and Samantha Chirunomula

8. RENAL
Kristi M. Schoeld

9. ENDOCRINE
Kristi M. Schoeld and Paul Opare-Addo

10. PERIOPERATIVE CONSIDERATIONS
David Araujo

Contributors

Seth Alkire, MD
Ventura County Medical Center Family Medicine Residency Program
Ventura, California
Chapter 4: Neurology
Chapter 7: Hematology

David Araujo, MD
Program Director, Ventura County Medical Center Family Medicine Residency Program
Associate Clinical Professor, UCLA David Geffen School of Medicine
Ventura, California
Chapter 1: Cardiovascular
Chapter 10: Perioperative Considerations

Samantha Chirunomula, MD
Ventura County Medical Center Family Medicine Residency Program
Ventura, California
Chapter 4: Neurology
Chapter 7: Hematology

Jacob A. David, MD, FAAFP
Associate Program Director
Ventura County Medical Center Family Medicine Residency Program
Clinical Instructor
UCLA David Geffen School of Medicine
Ventura, California
Chapter 1: Cardiovascular
Chapter 5: Gastroenterology
Chapter 11: Prevention of Complications

Neil Jorgensen, MD
Core Faculty, Ventura County Medical Center Family Medicine Residency Program
Ventura, California
Chapter 6: Infectious Disease

John Paul Kelada, MD
Ventura County Medical Center Family Medicine Residency Program
Ventura, California
Chapter 5: Gastroenterology

Tipu V. Khan, MD, FAAFP
Core Faculty, Ventura County Family Medicine Residency Program
Assistant Clinical Professor of Medicine, UCLA David Geffen School of Medicine
Ventura, California
Chapter 4: Neurology
Chapter 7: Hematology

Kristin H. King, MD
Ventura County Medical Center Family Medicine Residency Program
Ventura, California
Chapter 1: Cardiovascular

Marina Morie, MD
Ventura County Medical Center Family Medicine Residency Program
Ventura, California
Chapter 6: Infectious Disease

Heather Nennig, MD
Ventura County Medical Center Family Medicine Residency Program
Ventura, California
Chapter 12: End-of-Life Care

Paul Opare-Addo, MD, MPH
Ventura County Medical Center Family Medicine Residency Program
Ventura, California
Chapter 9: Endocrine

Leslie-Lynn Pawson, MD
Assistant Clinical Professor, Family Medicine, UCLA David Geffen School of Medicine
Core Faculty, Ventura County Medical Center Family Medicine Residency Program
Director of Palliative Care, Ventura County Medical Center
Ventura, California
Chapter 12: End-of-Life Care

Michael D. Ramirez, MD
Ventura County Medical Center Family Medicine Residency Program
Ventura, California
Chapter 1: Cardiovascular

James Rohlfing, MD
Ventura County Medical Center Family Medicine Residency Program
Ventura, California
Chapter 2: Vascular
Chapter 3: Pulmonary

Kristi M. Schoeld, MD
Assistant Clinical Professor of Medicine UCLA David Geffen School of Medicine
Core Faculty, Ventura County Medical Center Family Medicine Residency Program
Ventura, California
Chapter 8: Renal
Chapter 9: Endocrine
Chapter 11: Prevention of Complications

Zachary Zwolak, DO, FAAFP
Core Faculty, Ventura County Medical Center Family Medicine Residency Program
Clinical Instructor, UCLA David Geffen School of Medicine
Ventura, California
Chapter 2: Vascular
Chapter 3: Pulmonary

Preface

CURRENT: *Practice Guidelines in Inpatient Medicine, 2018–2019* digests evidence-based guidelines into salient point-of-care applications, enabling physicians, nurse practitioners, physician assistants, and medical students to incorporate the advice of major professional societies and government agencies into the care of hospitalized adults. Each section outlines the initial assessment, acute management, and subsequent care for conditions commonly encountered in the hospital, putting relevant information at the busy clinician's fingertips.

The author is grateful to the contributors, a select group of teaching faculty and resident physicians from the Ventura County Medical Center Family Medicine Residency Program, for conferring their expertise. Their knowledge of medicine and commitment to excellent care for all is inspiring, and will be the principal reason for any success the book enjoys.

Acutely ill patients deserve consistent, high-quality care informed by the guidelines summarized in CURRENT: *Practice Guidelines in Inpatient Medicine, 2018–2019*. However, no guideline encompasses every scenario, and no handbook obviates the need for clinical training and critical analysis of the available evidence. The clinician's experience and judgment and the patient's unique circumstances and preferences will at times supersede the recommendations found herein. Though painstaking efforts have been made to accurately represent these recommendations and to find and correct errors and omissions, inaccuracies may remain. If you care to suggest an improvement or correct an error, please e-mail at EditorialServices@mheducation.com.

Jacob A. David, MD, FAAFP

Cardiovascular

Jacob A. David
Michael D. Ramirez
Kristin H. King

ADULT LIFE SUPPORT

Adult Basic Life Support and Cardiopulmonary Resuscitation (CPR)

1. Unresponsive, no pulse, and not breathing
   a. Activate emergency response
   b. Obtain defibrillator; when available, attach and activate
   c. Begin CAB resuscitation (compressions, airway, breathing)
      i. Compressions: 100/min, 2 inches depth, allow recoil, minimize interruptions
      ii. Airway: Head tilt, chin lift; jaw thrust if trauma
      iii. Breathing: Compressions only; if second trained rescuer available, 30:2 ratio; with advanced airway, 8–10 breaths per minute
   d. Every 2 minutes, reassess, rotate compressors, and resume compressions promptly

Adult Advanced Cardiac Life Support

1. Cardiac arrest
   a. Activate emergency response
   b. Begin CPR while obtaining rhythm assessment
   c. Non-shockable rhythm (asystole, pulseless electrical activity)
      i. CPR 2-minute cycles
      ii. Give epinephrine every 3–5 minutes
      iii. Reassess for shockable rhythm at end of each CPR cycle
      iv. Treat reversible causes
   d. Shockable rhythm (ventricular fibrillation, pulseless ventricular tachycardia)
   e. Shock
   f. Resume CPR immediately, 2-minute cycles
   g. Reassess for shockable rhythm at end of each CPR cycle; shock if appropriate

    h. Give epinephrine every 3–5 minutes

    i. Consider amiodarone or lidocaine if no ROSC after epinephrine and shock

    j. Treat reversible causes

2. ROSC: Begin postarrest care

Source:

1. Neumar RW, Shuster M, Callaway CW, et al. Part 1: Executive summary. 2015 American Heart Association guidelines update for cardiopulmonary resuscitation and emergency cardiovascular care. Circulation. 2015;132 (18 Suppl 2):S315–S367. [http://circ.ahajournals.org/content/132/18_suppl_2/S315]

ST-ELEVATION MYOCARDIAL INFARCTION

Initial Assessment (ESC 2012)

1. Draw serum markers routinely, but do not wait for results to initiate reperfusion therapy

Acute Medical Management

1. Antiplatelet therapy (ACC/AHA 2013, ESC 2012, NICE 2013)

    a. Give aspirin (162–325 mg) at presentation

    b. If treating with PCI, give a loading dose of an ADP-receptor inhibitor (clopidogrel[1] 600 mg, prasugrel[1] 60 mg, or ticagrelor 180 mg)[2] as early as possible

    c. If treating with fibrinolytics, give a loading dose of clopidogrel (300 mg; 75 mg if >75 years of age) with aspirin

2. Beta blockers

    a. ACC/AHA: If hypertensive or having ongoing ischemia, give beta blocker at time of presentation, unless contraindicated

3. Oxygen

    a. ESC: Give supplemental oxygen to treat hypoxia (SaO_2 <95%), breathlessness, or acute heart failure

4. Analgesics

    a. ESC: Give IV opioids to relieve pain

5. Anticoagulation (ACC/AHA 2013, ESC 2012, NICE 2013)

    a. If patient will receive primary PCI, give anticoagulation with unfractionated heparin (UFH), enoxaparin, or bivalirudin[3]; a glycoprotein IIb/IIIa inhibitor (abciximab, eptifibatide, tirofiban) may be added to UFH

---

[1]Do not administer prasugrel to patients with a history of prior stroke or TIA.

[2]ESC guidelines favor prasugrel or ticagrelor over clopidogrel. ACC/AHA does not state a preference.

[3]ESC guidelines favor bivalirudin or enoxaparin to unfractionated heparin. ACC/AHA does not state a preference.

b. If patient will receive fibrinolytics, give anticoagulation until hospital discharge (minimum 48 hours, up to 8 days) or until revascularization is performed; options include UFH (titrated to a PTT of 1.5–2.0 times control), enoxaparin (IV bolus followed in 15 minutes by subcutaneous injection), or fondaparinux (initial IV dose followed in 24 hours by subcutaneous therapy)

Coronary Reperfusion Therapy

1. PCI (ACC/AHA 2013, ESC 2012, NICE 2013)
   a. Initiate reperfusion therapy (PCI, if experienced operators are available in a timely fashion) to all eligible patients within 12 hours of symptom onset; it remains beneficial up to at least 24 hours if there is evidence of ongoing ischemia
   b. Primary PCI is preferable to fibrinolysis if performed by an experienced team within 120 minutes of first medical contact
   c. Primary PCI is indicated in all patients with STEMI and cardiogenic shock or severe acute heart failure
   d. In PCI for STEMI, use either a bare-metal or drug-eluting stent; use a bare-metal stent in patients with high bleeding risk, inability to comply with 1 year of dual antiplatelet therapy, or upcoming invasive procedure
   e. In comatose patients, use therapeutic hypothermia
2. Fibrinolytic therapy (ACC/AHA 2013, ESC 2012, NICE 2013)
   a. If timely PCI is not available, give fibrinolytic therapy within 30 minutes of hospital arrival, unless contraindicated; it is most useful if ischemic symptoms started within the past 12 hours, and is a reasonable choice between 12 and 24 hours if there is evidence of ongoing ischemia or a large area of myocardium at risk
   b. Transfer to PCI-capable center
   c. ACC/AHA: Transfer for urgent PCI if fibrinolysis fails
   d. ESC: Transfer all patients after fibrinolysis; rescue PCI is indicated immediately when fibrinolysis has failed

Management After Stabilization

1. Antiplatelet therapy (ACC/AHA 2016, ESC 2012)
   a. Continue aspirin 81 mg indefinitely
   b. After PCI for ACS, give dual antiplatelet therapy[4] for 1 year
      i. ESC: "Up to 12 months," with strict minimum of 1 month for bare-metal stent and 6 months for drug-eluting stent
      ii. ACC/AHA: "Discontinuation after 6 months may be reasonable" if high bleeding risk; ">1 year may be reasonable" if low bleeding risk
   c. After fibrinolytic therapy, continue dual antiplatelet therapy for at least 14 days and up to 1 year

---

[4]ESC guidelines favor prasugrel or ticagrelor over clopidogrel for dual antiplatelet therapy. ACC/AHA lists three options: clopidogrel 75 mg daily, prasugrel 10 mg daily, or ticagrelor 90 mg BID.

d. ESC: If anticoagulation is otherwise indicated (i.e., for atrial fibrillation (AF)), give it in addition to antiplatelet therapy

2. Beta blockers (ACC/AHA 2013, ESC 2012)

   a. Initiate oral beta blockers in the first 24 hours, unless heart failure, evidence of a low output state, or other contraindications

3. Renin-angiotensin-aldosterone system inhibitors (ACC/AHA 2013, ESC 2012)

   a. Administer ACE inhibitor (or angiotensin receptor blocker, if intolerant of ACE) within the first 24 hours if anterior infarction, heart failure, or ejection fraction ≤40%

   b. Give an aldosterone antagonist to patients who are already receiving an ACE inhibitor and beta blocker, and whose ejection fraction is ≤40% and either have symptomatic heart failure or diabetes mellitus, unless contraindicated

4. Lipid-lowering agents (ACC/AHA 2013, ESC 2012)

   a. Start or continue high-intensity statin therapy, unless contraindicated

   b. Obtain a fasting lipid panel; ESC: Remeasure LDL after 1 month to ensure LDL <70 mg/dL

5. Implantable cardioverter-defibrillator therapy (ACC/AHA 2013, ESC 2012)

   a. ICD therapy is indicated before discharge in patients who develop sustained VT/VF more than 48 hours after STEMI, unless the arrhythmia is due to ischemia, reinfarction, or metabolic abnormalities

   b. If LVEF is initially reduced, reevaluate LVEF to assess candidacy for ICD therapy

6. Post-ACS risk assessments (ACC/AHA 2013, ESC 2012)

   a. If patient did not undergo coronary angiography, or in patients with multi-vessel disease, perform noninvasive testing for ischemia before discharge

Sources:

1. ACC/AHA 2013: O'Gara PT, Kushner FG, Ascheim DD, et al. 2013 ACCF/AHA guideline for the management of ST-elevation myocardial infarction. J Am Coll Cardiol. 2013 Jan 29;61(4). [https://www.guideline.gov/summaries/summary/39429?]

2. ESC 2012: Steg PG, James SK, Atar D, et al. ESC guidelines for the management of acute myocardial infarction in patients presenting with ST-segment elevation. Eur Heart J. 2012 Oct;33(20):2569–2619. [https://www.guideline.gov/summaries/summary/39353?]

3. NICE 2013: National Clinical Guideline Centre. Myocardial infarction with ST-segment elevation. The acute management of myocardial infarction with ST-segment elevation. National Institute for Health and Care Excellence (NICE); 2013 Jul. 28 p. [https://www.guideline.gov/summaries/summary/47019?]

4. ACC/AHA 2016: Levine GN, Bates ER, Bittl JA, et al. 2016 ACC/AHA guideline focused update on duration of dual antiplatelet therapy in patients with coronary artery disease. Am Coll Cardiol. 2016;68(10):1082–1115. [http://content.onlinejacc.org/article.aspx?articleid=2507082]

NON-ST-ELEVATION MYOCARDIAL INFARCTION

Initial Assessment (ACC/AHA 2014)

1. If ACS is suspected, perform an EKG within 10 minutes; if initial EKG is non-diagnostic, repeat q15–30 minutes during the first hour
2. Trend cardiac troponin I or T levels at symptom onset and 3–6 hours later; draw additional levels beyond 6 hours if EKG or clinical presentation suggest a high probability of ACS
3. Assess prognosis with risk scores
   a. TIMI risk score
      i. Predicts 30-day and 1-year mortality in ACS (mortality rises at TIMI = 3–4)
      ii. 1 point each for:
         1. Age ≥65
         2. ≥3 risk factors for CAD[5]
         3. Known CAD
         4. ST changes on EKG (≥0.5 mm)
         5. Active angina (≥2 episodes in past 24 hours)
         6. Aspirin in past 7 days
         7. Elevated cardiac marker
   b. GRACE risk model
      i. Predicts in-hospital and post-discharge mortality or MI
      ii. Downloadable tool: [http://www.outcomes-umassmed.org/grace/]
   c. ACR appropriateness criteria for cardiac imaging (ACR 2014)
      i. Usually appropriate to order
         1. Myocardial perfusion imaging (MPI) (rest and stress) or coronary angiogram, if intermediate to high likelihood for CAD
         2. Rest-only MPI has good negative predictive value
         3. Consider stress echo if resting echo and cardiac enzymes are normal
      ii. Usually not appropriate to order:
         1. MRI heart – Primarily useful to rule out aortic dissection
         2. Transesophageal echocardiogram – Contraindicated in ACS
         3. CT coronary calcium – Not useful in acute settings
         4. MRA coronaries – Technically difficult, no validated protocols

[5]Risk factors for CAD: FamHx CAD, HTN, dyslipidemia, DM, smoking.

CHAPTER 1

Acute Medical Management (ACC/AHA 2014)

1. Antiplatelet therapy
   a. Give dual antiplatelet therapy in likely or definite NSTE-ACS
      i. Aspirin (162–325 mg, non-enteric-coated) immediately
      ii. Clopidogrel (300–600 mg loading dose, then maintenance) or ticagrelor (180 mg loading dose, then maintenance)[6]
2. Anticoagulation
   a. Anticoagulate, in addition to dual antiplatelet therapy[7]
   b. Use UFH, enoxaparin, or fondaparinux; strongest evidence supports enoxaparin
3. Beta blockers
   a. Give oral beta blockers in the first 24 hours, unless signs of heart failure, low output state, risk factors for cardiogenic shock, or other contraindications to beta blockade[8]
   b. If stable reduced LVEF HF, continue long-acting metoprolol succinate, carvedilol, or bisoprolol
   c. In patients already on beta blockers, continue them if LVEF is normal
4. Renin-angiotensin-aldosterone system inhibitors: Start ACE inhibitor
5. Lipid-lowering agents: Start or continue high-intensity statin, unless contraindicated
6. Nitrates
   a. Give sublingual nitroglycerin q5 min × 3 for ongoing ischemic pain
   b. Use IV nitroglycerin for persistent ischemia, heart failure, or hypertension[9]
7. Calcium channel blockers: Use non-dihydropyridine calcium channel blockers as initial therapy if beta blockers are contraindicated, or for recurrent ischemia despite beta blocker and nitrate use[10]
8. Oxygen: Supplemental oxygen if SaO_2 ≤90% or respiratory distress
9. Analgesics
   a. IV morphine is appropriate if anti-ischemic medications have been maximized
   b. Do not give NSAIDs

---

[6]Ticagrelor lowers mortality rate slightly more than clopidogrel, but had more adverse effects (dyspnea, bradycardia) and is dosed more frequently.

[7]Compared with aspirin, heparin reduces occurrence of MI (NNT 33) but does not reduce mortality, need for revascularization, or recurrent angina. NNH for bleeding is 17 (Cochrane Database Syst Rev. 2008;2:CD003462).

[8]Beta blockers are contraindicated if PR interval >0.24 seconds, second- or third-degree heart block without pacemaker, active asthma, or reactive airway disease.

[9]Nitrates are contraindicated if a phosphodiesterase inhibitor was recently used.

[10]Contraindications to calcium channel blockers in NSTE-ACS include LV dysfunction, risk for cardiogenic shock, prolonged PR interval, or second- or third-degree AV block without a pacemaker.

TABLE 1-1

DUAL ANTIPLATELET THERAPY DURATION AFTER ACUTE CORONARY SYNDROME		
Acute ACS Treatment	**Second Antiplatelet Agent**	**Duration of DAPT**
Medical therapy	Clopidogrel or ticagrelor	12 months, "at least"
Thrombolytics for STEMI	Clopidogrel	14 days minimum
		Ideally, 12 months "at least"
PCI (drug-eluding or bare-metal stent)	Clopidogrel, prasugrel, or ticagrelor	12 months, "at least"
CABG	P2Y12 inhibitor	Complete 1 year of dual therapy

Source: Adapted from ACC/AHA 2016.

Interventions
1. Coronary reperfusion therapy (ACC/AHA 2013)
   a. Do not give fibrinolytic therapy for non-ST-elevation MIs

Management After Stabilization (ACC/AHA 2014)
1. Antiplatelet therapy
   a. Continue aspirin (81–325 mg/day) indefinitely
   b. If unable to take aspirin, give clopidogrel 75 mg daily
   c. Dual antiplatelet therapy (clopidogrel or ticagrelor in addition to aspirin)
      i. "Up to" 12 months if not stented
      ii. "At least" 12 months if stented
      iii. See Table 1-1 for more detail
2. Beta blockers
3. Renin-angiotensin-aldosterone system inhibitors
   a. Start ACE inhibitors (or ARB, if ACE-intolerant) and continue indefinitely (unless contraindicated) if any of the following:
      i. LVEF <0.40
      ii. HTN
      iii. DM
      iv. Stable CKD
   b. Aldosterone blockade (i.e., spironolactone) in patients meeting all the following criteria:
      i. Adequate kidney function[11] and potassium level[12]
      ii. Receiving therapeutic doses of ACE inhibitor and beta blocker
      iii. LVEF ≤0.40, diabetes mellitus, or clinical heart failure

[11]Cr ≤2.5 mg/dL in men or ≤2.0 mg/dL in women.
[12]K+ ≤5.0 mEq/L.

4. Lipid-lowering agents: Start/continue high-intensity statin, unless contraindicated

Sources:

1. ACC/AHA 2013: O'Gara PT, Kushner FG, Ascheim DD, et al. 2013 ACCF/AHA guideline for the management of ST-elevation myocardial infarction. J Am Coll Cardiol. 2013 Jan 29;61(4). [https://www.guideline .gov/summaries/summary/39429?]
2. ACC/AHA 2014: Amsteradm EA, Wenger NK, Brindis RG, et al. 2014 AHA/ACC guideline for the management of patients with non-ST-elevation acute coronary syndromes. J Am Coll Cardiol. 2014;64(24):e139–e228. [http://content.onlinejacc.org/article.aspx?articleid=1910086]
3. ACR 2014: Mammen L, Abbara S, Dorbala S. ACR Appropriateness Criteria® chest pain suggestive of acute coronary syndrome. American College of Radiology (ACR); 2014. 10 p. [https://guidelines.gov/ summaries/summary/48280]
4. ACC/AHA 2016: Levine GN, Bates ER, Bittl JA, et al. 2016 ACC/AHA guideline focused update on duration of dual antiplatelet therapy in patients with coronary artery disease. Am Coll Cardiol. 2016;68(10):1082–1115. [http://content.onlinejacc.org/article.aspx?articleid=2507082]

CONGESTIVE HEART FAILURE

Initial Assessment (ACC/AHA 2013, ESC 2012)

1. Assess volume status clinically: Weight, jugular venous pressure (JVP), orthopnea, edema
2. Initial laboratory evaluation[13]
   a. CBCD (ESC: Rule out anemia as alternative cause)
   b. UAUM
   c. Serum electrolytes including Ca^{++}, Mg^{++}
   d. BUN/Cr
   e. Glucose
   f. Fasting lipid profile
   g. Liver function test (LFT)
   h. Thyroid-stimulating hormone (TSH)
3. Biomarkers
   a. Brain natriuretic peptide (BNP) or NT-proBNP
      i. Supports clinical judgment for diagnosis of acutely decompensated HF
      ii. Useful in establishing prognosis and disease severity
      iii. Serial measurement or BNP-guided therapy is NOT well established

---

[13] ACC/AHA: Assess for end-organ damage.

    b. Troponin-I

        i. ACC/AHA: Rule out ACS precipitating acute HF decompensation immediately, including EKG evaluation

4. Noninvasive cardiac imaging

    a. Chest X-ray in any patient with new onset HT or acute decompensation

        i. Assess heart size and pulmonary congestion

        ii. Rule out other etiologies that may be contributing to symptoms

    b. EKG as above to rule out ACS precipitating decompensation

    c. 2D ECHO with Doppler to assess ventricular function, size, wall thickness, wall motion, valve function

        i. Initial evaluation of patients presenting with HF

        ii. Known HF in patient with

            1. Significant change in clinical status

            2. Recovered from clinical event

            3. Underwent treatment that may impact/improve cardiac function

        iii. NO benefit in routine reevaluation of LV function if no clinical change

    d. Myocardial perfusion scan with stress test (exercise or medical) in patients who present for initial evaluation OR with known CAD and no angina

5. Invasive cardiac monitoring

    a. NO benefit in acute decompensation if normotensive and symptomatic improvement with diuretics and vasodilators

    b. Pulmonary artery catheter: If intracardiac filling pressures cannot be determined on clinical assessment and patient has significant dyspnea, consider PAWP to guide therapy

    c. Coronary arteriography: Use when ischemia may be contributing to decompensation

6. Stage severity of heart failure for chronic therapy decision making

    a. ACC/AHA

        i. Stage A: At risk for HF, without structural heart disease and asymptomatic

        ii. Stage B: Evidence of structural heart disease (i.e., reduced ejection fraction, left ventricular hypertrophy, chamber enlargement) who have not yet developed symptoms of heart failure

        iii. Stage C: Structural heart disease WITH symptoms of HF

        iv. Stage D: Refractory disease requiring advanced intervention, including BiV pacemaker, IVAD, transplant

    b. NYHA

        i. No limitation of physical activity; ordinary physical activity does not cause fatigue, palpitations, dyspnea

    ii. Slight limitation of physical activity; asymptomatic at rest, but ordinary physical activity causes symptoms

    iii. Marked limitation with physical activity, remains asymptomatic at rest

    iv. Unable to carry on any physical activity; symptomatic at rest

Acute Medical Management (ACC/AHA 2013)

1. Maintenance of guideline-directed medical therapy
   a. Continue guideline-directed medical therapy in the absence of hemodynamic instability
      i. Decrease beta blocker by 50% if moderate heart failure
      ii. Discontinue beta blocker if severe symptoms or hypotensive
      iii. Consider transition of ACEI/ARB to hydralazine/nitrates in AKI
   b. Start beta blocker once volume status is optimized to baseline and patient is no longer receiving IV diuretics, vasodilators, or inotropic agents; start at low dose and only when patients are stable clinically
2. Diuresis
   a. Start loop diuretic promptly
   b. Start at 20–40 mg IV once if no prior therapy; may repeat same dose or increase by 20 mg and administer 1–2 hours after initial dose and titrate to desired UOP and clinical effect (maximum 200 mg/day)
   c. If on chronic diuretic therapy, increase TDD by 2× PO home dose with intermittent boluses or with furosemide drip[14]
   d. Assess UOP and clinical respiratory status; adjust diuretic dose to relieve symptoms, reduce volume excess, and avoid hypotension
   e. Check daily serum electrolytes and Cr/BUN while on diuretic therapy
   f. Daily weights, strict input/output measurements daily
   g. If inadequate diuresis, can add a thiazide diuretic to improve diuresis
3. IV vasodilators
   a. Consider nitroglycerin, nitroprusside, or nesiritide to reduce dyspneic symptoms, in addition to diuretics
   b. Do not use if symptomatic hypotension
4. Inotropes
   a. Consider low-dose dopamine infusion in setting of hypotension and poor cardiac output
   b. Beneficial for inotropic improvement
   c. Helps to improve diuresis and prevent AKI by improving renal blood flow
5. Ultrafiltration
   a. Used in cases of refractory congestion unresponsive to medical therapy
   b. Increases risk of progression to renal failure (NEJM. 2012;367:2296)

---

[14]No significant change in mortality with drip versus bolus.

Management After Stabilization (ACC/AHA 2013, ESC 2012)

1. See Table 1-2 for indications for various interventions
2. Stage A: At risk of HF (HTN, FHx of cardiomyopathy) but asymptomatic and no structural heart disease
   a. Treat HTN, lipid disorders, DMII
   b. ACEI/ARB if HTN, DM, PAD, CAD
   c. Stop smoking; limit alcohol use
   d. Increase exercise and low sodium (<2 g/day) diet, avoid/treat obesity

TABLE 1-2

INTERVENTIONS FOR MANAGEMENT OF CHRONIC HEART FAILURE		
Intervention	**Data**	**Indication**
Lifestyle modifications	Sodium goal <2 g/day; exercising training; cessation of smoking; limit alcohol use; treat/avoid obesity	NYHA Stages A–D
Angiotensin-converting enzyme inhibitor (ACEI)	Can decrease mortality by 40%; side effects of cough and angioedema	NYHA Stages A–D
Angiotensin receptor blocker (ARB)	Alternative to ACEI if unable to tolerate; equally effective as ACEI	NYHA Stages A–D
Beta blocker	Carvedilol, bisoprolol, metoprolol; improvement in mortality and decreased hospitalizations; may make symptoms worse initially due to decreased EF	NYHA Stages B–D
Aldosterone receptor antagonist	NYHA II–IV and EF <35%; do NOT use if hyperkalemic or Cr >2.5; decreases mortality in this subset of patients	NYHA Stages C–D
Hydralazine and isosorbide dinitrate	Suitable replacement of ACEI/ARB to decrease mortality if not tolerated due to renal dysfunction	NYHA Stages C–D Unable to tolerate ACEI/ARB
Digoxin	No change in mortality; improved symptoms and decreased hospitalizations if EF <45%	NYHA Stages C–D Reduced EF <45%
Diuretics	No change in mortality; improved symptoms and decreased hospitalizations	NYHA Stages C–D

Source: Adapted from AHA/ACC 2013 and ESC 2012.

3. Stage B: Structural heart disease, but remains asymptomatic
   a. As per Stage A treatment; use ACEI/ARB to prevent symptomatic HF/progression
   b. Add evidence-based beta blocker if MI/CAD or decreased EF (bisoprolol, carvedilol, or metoprolol)
   c. If asymptomatic ischemic cardiomyopathy less than 40 days post-MI, EF <30%, on all GDMT, and greater than 1 year expected survival implantable cardioverter-defibrillator is reasonable to prevent sudden death
      i. ACC/AHA: AVOID non-dihydropyridine CCBs with negative inotropic effects
4. Stage C: Structural changes and any history of symptoms of HF
   a. Non-pharmacologic intervention
      i. Low-sodium diet to prevent exacerbations and congestion
      ii. CPAP if HF + sleep apnea
      iii. Exercise training and cardiac rehabilitation
   b. Continue all pharmacologic interventions for Stages A and B
      i. ACEI: In all patients with reduced ejection fraction
         1. ARB if ACEI cannot be tolerated by patient
         2. ARBs are near equally efficacious to reduce morbidity and mortality as ACEI
         3. Avoid combined use of ACEI, ARB, and aldosterone antagonist
      ii. Beta blocker: Patients with reduced EF and any history of symptoms (carvedilol, bisoprolol, metoprolol)
      iii. Aldosterone receptor antagonists (mineralocorticoid receptor antagonists): Give to patients with NYHA II–IV and EF <35% OR in acute MI patients with EF <40% with symptoms of HF and/or DM
         1. Cr 2.5 mg/dL or less in men, 2.0 mg/dL in women
         2. Potassium less than 5.0 mEq/L
         3. Carefully monitor potassium, renal function
      iv. Hydralazine and isosorbide dinitrate: Can be substituted if ACEI/ARB is not tolerated due to side effects, hypotension, renal insufficiency
      v. Digoxin: Beneficial in patients with reduced EF to decrease hospitalizations, however, no change in mortality
         1. ESC: EF <45% who cannot tolerate a beta blocker; consider amiodarone if unable to tolerate beta blocker nor digoxin
         2. Optimal digoxin level 0.5–0.8 ng/mL (JAMA. 2003;289:871)
      vi. Do not anticoagulate patients with chronic HFrEF without AF or prior VTE; consider anticoagulation in patients with AF
      vii. Statins are NOT beneficial as adjunctive therapy if solely prescribed for diagnosis of heart failure in the absence of hyperlipidemia

viii. AVOID calcium channel blocking drugs as they can precipitate exacerbations and increase morbidity and mortality

c. Add diuretic

    i. Start furosemide in patients with any evidence of fluid retention to reduce symptoms of dyspnea and fluid overload; start at 20 mg PO daily and monitor UOP/Cr and symptoms

    ii. Implantable cardioverter-defibrillator for primary prevention of cardiac death

    iii. ACC/AHA: Non-ischemic dilated cardiomyopathy or ischemic heart disease at least 40 days post-MI with LVEF <35% and NYHA II–IV symptoms

    iv. Cardiac resynchronization therapy (CRT)

        1. ACC/AHA, ESC: LVEF <35%, sinus rhythm, LBBB with QRS >150 ms, NYHA II

        2. ESC: LVEF <30%, sinus rhythm, non-LBBB QRS >150 ms

        3. ACC/AHA: LVEF <35%, AF requiring ventricular pacing and AV node ablation or pharmacologic suppression of AV node will allow near 100% of ventricular pacing with CRT

        4. Do not use with NYHA I–II symptoms and non-LBBB with QRS <150 ms

5. Stage D: Refractory HF requiring specialized interventions

  a. Water restriction: 1.5–2 L/day to reduce fluid overload

  b. Inotropic support: Start intravenous inotropic support to maintain system perfusion and end-organ perfusion until resolution of acute exacerbation OR until definitive therapy (coronary revascularization, heart transplant)

    i. Do not use long term unless specific indication for perfusion as above, or for palliative care

    ii. Do not use unless evidence of severe systolic dysfunction, hypotension, or impaired perfusion

  c. Mechanical circulatory support

    i. Beneficial only if definitive management with cardiac transplantation is anticipated or cardiac recovery is expected; use only as bridge to recovery with transplant or bridge to decision in profound hemodynamic compromise

  d. Cardiac transplantation: Indicated for Stage D HF despite GDMT, ICD/CRT device, and surgical management

6. ACC/AHA: Heart failure with preserved EF

  a. Diuresis

  b. Blood pressure control

  c. No benefit found with ACEI/ARB

  d. Aldosterone antagonist may reduce hospitalizations and mortality

Sources:

1. ACC/AHA 2013: Yancy CW, Jessup M, Bozkurt B, et al. 2013 ACCF/AHA guideline for the management of heart failure. Circulation. 2013; CIR.0b013e31829e8776. [http://circ.ahajournals.org/content/early/2013/06/03/CIR.0b013e31829e8776]

2. ESC 2012: McMurray JJ, Adamopoulos S, Anker SD, et al. ESC guidelines for the diagnosis and treatment of acute and chronic heart failure 2012. Eur J Heart Fail. 2012;14(8):803–869. [https://www.ncbi.nlm.nih.gov/pubmed/22828712]

3. Bart BA, Goldsmith SR, Lee KL, et al. Ultrafiltration in decompensated heart failure with cardiorenal syndrome. NEJM. 2012;367(24):2296–3304. [https://www.ncbi.nlm.nih.gov/pubmed/23131078]

4. Rathore, SS, Curtis JP, Want Y, et al. Association of serum digoxin concentration and outcomes in patients with heart failure. JAMA. 2003;289(7):871–878. [https://www.ncbi.nlm.nih.gov/pubmed/12588271]

ATRIAL FIBRILLATION

Initial Assessment (ACC/AHA 2014, NICE 2014)

1. History
   a. Determine whether paroxysmal, persistent, long-standing persistent, or permanent
   b. Obtain symptoms, prior treatment, family history, and review of reversible risk factors
   c. Specifically assess for dyspnea, palpitations, breathlessness, chest discomfort, stroke
2. Physical exam: Identify irregular pulse, irregular jugular venous pulse
3. Noninvasive cardiac imaging
   a. Get EKG to confirm irregular pulse and confirm AF
   b. NICE: Transthoracic ECHO
      i. As a baseline for long-term management
      ii. If high risk or suspicion of underlying structural disease (CHF, murmur)
      iii. To refine clinical risk stratification for anticoagulation
      iv. Do not perform TTE to further stratify stroke risk if anticoagulation therapy is planned
   c. Perform transesophageal ECHO when
      i. TTE demonstrates valvular disease or vegetation
      ii. TTE is technically difficult with poor quality and cardiac abnormalities must be excluded

    d. ACC/AHA: Electrophysiological study

        i. If AF is secondary to supraventricular tachycardia, such as AVNRT or multifocal atrial tachycardia (MAT), ablation may prevent and/or reduce recurrence of AF

    e. Prolonged rhythm monitoring is necessary to identify asymptomatic episodes

        i. Holter monitor, telemetry, auto-triggered event recorder

    f. NICE: Exercise stress test can assess adequacy of rate control

    g. NICE: Sleep study is beneficial if sleep apnea is expected

4. Laboratory evaluation

    a. NICE: BNP or NT-proBNP may be elevated in patients with paroxysmal/persistent AF in the absence of CHF, and normalize rapidly with cardioversion to sinus rhythm

Acute Medical Management

1. New or recent onset AF (AHA/ACC 2014, NICE 2014)

    a. Unstable: Any hemodynamic instability: Hypotensive, tachypneic, rapid ventricular response with symptoms

        i. Immediate cardioversion regardless of anticoagulation status; do not delay cardioversion for anticoagulation

        ii. Also indicated if refractory RVR despite medical therapy with ongoing ischemia, hypotension, or HF

    b. Stable (normotensive, asymptomatic): Start with rate control

        i. NICE: Offer rate control as the first-line strategy unless

            1. AF has a reversible cause

            2. Heart failure thought to be primarily caused by AF

            3. New-onset AF

            4. Atrial flutter whose condition is considered suitable for an ablation strategy to restore sinus rhythm

            5. A rhythm control strategy would be more suitable based on clinical judgement

        ii. HR targets in rate control (Lancet. 2016;388:818)

            1. If any symptoms: HR <80

            2. If asymptomatic, EF >40%: Goal HR >110

        iii. Start rate control with beta blocker or calcium channel blocker

            1. Diltiazem

                a. Acute: 0.25 mg/kg IV over 2 minutes, then repeat in 30 minutes if heart rate remains above goal

                b. Maintenance: 120–360 mg/day PO divided QID

                    i. Preferred in severe COPD cases as will not exacerbate bronchoconstriction as beta blocker may

2. Metoprolol tartrate
   a. Acute: 2.5–5 mg IV over 2 minutes, then repeat every 5 minutes up to additional 3 doses
   b. Maintenance: 25–100 mg PO BID/TID
      i. Can decrease blood pressure, worsen bronchospasm, and exacerbate HF
      ii. Preferred if known coronary artery disease
3. NICE: If monotherapy does not control symptoms, and if continuing symptoms are due to poor ventricular rate control, consider combination therapy with any two of the following:
   a. Beta blocker
   b. Diltiazem
   c. Digoxin

Interventions (AHA/ACC 2014, NICE 2014)

1. Nonurgent cardioversion, electrical and pharmacologic: Use to restore sinus rhythm once stable with no hemodynamic compromise
   a. ACC/AHA: Consider admission for cardioversion acutely if <48 hours from onset, 1st episode, and low stroke risk
      i. Anticoagulate with UFH IV, then bridge to oral anticoagulation for at least 4 weeks post cardioversion
      ii. Thromboembolic risk is highest in first 72 hours after cardioversion and majority of events occur within 10 days
   b. If in AF >48 hours, there is a 2%–5% risk of stroke
      i. Therapeutic anticoagulation for at least 3 weeks is required prior to cardioversion
      ii. Or, can obtain TEE to rule out thrombus
         1. If TEE negative can perform cardioversion without waiting 3 weeks
         2. If TEE positive, anticoagulate for at least 3 weeks
   c. Anticoagulation after cardioversion: 4 weeks minimum
   d. Antiarrhythmic pretreatment for electrical cardioversion: Can consider class III or class IC antiarrhythmic drug, particularly if first attempt failed to convert
      i. NICE: Consider amiodarone therapy starting 4 weeks before and continuing for up to 12 months after electrical cardioversion to maintain sinus rhythm

Management After Stabilization

1. Start anticoagulation once rate controlled (AHA/ACC 2014, NICE 2014)
   a. Assess stroke and bleeding risk
      i. Use CHA2DS2-VASc and HAS-BLED scores to individualize decision to start anticoagulation in patients with nonvalvular AF (including paroxysmal, persistent, or permanent AF and atrial flutter)

      ii. Use CHA2DS2-VASc stroke risk score to assess stroke risk

        1. If 2 or greater, start anticoagulation

        2. If 1, consider anticoagulation and discuss with patient

        3. If 0, do not start anticoagulation

      iii. Use HAS-BLED score to assess bleed risk

        1. Offer modification to anticoagulation regimen and monitoring in the following cases:

          a. If HAS-BLED score is 3 or greater

          b. Uncontrolled hypertension

          c. Poor control of INR

          d. NSAID/Aspirin concomitant use

          e. Harmful alcohol consumption

  b. Choice of anticoagulant: NOAC (nonvalvular AF only) or warfarin

    i. Warfarin (vitamin K antagonist (VKA)): Start most patients with 5 mg PO daily × 2 days then check INR and titrate per institutional algorithm; INR goal of 2–3

      1. AHA/ACC: Choose warfarin over NOACs if ESRD (CrCl <15 mL/min) or on hemodialysis

    ii. Dabigatran (direct thrombin inhibitor)[15]: 150 mg PO BID; if CrCl 15–30 mL/min, 75 mg PO BID

    iii. Rivaroxaban (FXa inhibitor): 20 mg PO daily with dinner

    iv. Apixaban (FXa inhibitor): 5 mg PO BID

    v. Edoxaban (FXa inhibitor): 60 mg PO daily

    vi. ASA + clopidogrel: Consider if patient declines anticoagulation therapy; improves stroke mortality overall, albeit less than anticoagulation

  c. Choice of antiarrhythmic (AHA/ACC 2014)[16]

    i. Class III

      1. Ibutilide: IV infusion of 1 mg over 10 minutes, then repeated once if unsuccessful

        a. ACC/AHA: Highest percentage of success (~50%) if initiated within 7 days of onset

        b. Contraindicated if hypokalemic or prolonged QT

        c. Give with magnesium IV

      2. Amiodarone: 150 mg IV over 10 minutes, then 1 mg/min for 6 hours, then 0.5 mg/min for 18 hours or switch to PO, with 200–400 mg daily for maintenance

        a. Oral: 600–800 mg daily in divided doses to a total load of up to 10 g, then 200–400 mg QD as maintenance

---

[15] Increased GI bleeding risk with dabigatran versus other agents.
[16] Antiarrhythmic drugs do not decrease mortality or stroke risk compared to rate control.

    i. Amiodarone PO is the most successful drug in maintaining sinus rhythm

    ii. Can cause marked bradycardia and prolong QT

    iii. Safest in AF with structural heart disease

      3. Dofetilide: 500 mcg PO BID if CrCl >60; adjust dosing if CKD

  d. Class IC

    i. Flecainide: 300 mg PO once for conversion, then 150 mg BID for maintenance

    ii. Propafenone: 600 mg PO once for conversion, then 300 mg TID for maintenance

      1. For both medications

        a. Do not use if structural or ischemic heart disease (pro-arrhythmic)

        b. Pretreat with AV node blocker to prevent conversion to atrial flutter with 1:1 AV conduction

Sources:

1. ACC/AHA 2014. January CT, Wann LS, Alpert JS, et al. 2014 AHA/ACC/HRS guideline for the management of patients with atrial fibrillation. Circulation. 2014;CIR.0000000000000041. [http://circ.ahajournals.org/content/early/2014/04/10/CIR.0000000000000041]

2. NICE 2014: National Clinical Guideline Centre. Atrial fibrillation: the management of atrial fibrillation. London (UK): National Institute for Health and Care Excellence (NICE); 2014. 49 p. (Clinical guideline; no. 180). [http://www.guideline.gov/content.aspx?id=48333]

3. Van Gelder IC, Rienstra M, Crijns HJ, Olshansky B. Rate control in atrial fibrillation. Lancet. 2016;388:818–828. [https://www.ncbi.nlm.nih.gov/pubmed/27560277]

SUPRAVENTRICULAR TACHYCARDIA

Initial Assessment (AHA/ACC/HRS 2015)

1. Definition and diagnosis

  a. Supraventricular tachycardia (SVT) includes any arrhythmia that originates at or above the bundle of His; excluding AF, as it is considered its own distinct arrhythmia

  b. QRS is typically narrow, except in cases of AV node dysfunction or pre-excitation syndromes from accessory pathways, as described below

  c. For any symptoms of palpitations, start with 12-lead ECG

  d. If prior palpitations, consider EKG to identify pre-excitation syndrome which would require urgent evaluation with electrophysiology

2. Types of SVT (NEJM. 2012;367:1438)

  a. Sinus tachycardia

b. Most common SVT, and is not typically pathologic, but rather a physiologic response to a stressor

c. The rate is regular and rarely exceeds 220

d. Upright P waves in leads I, II

e. P waves precede every QRS

3. Atrial flutter

a. Second most common pathologic arrhythmia behind AF; caused by reentrant circuit around tricuspid valve in right atrium

b. Organized regular rhythm

c. Atrial rate of ~280–300 beats per minute with 2:1 AV nodal conduction

d. This results in ventricular rate of ~150 beats per minute

e. Flutter waves can often be obscured by T waves at this rate, however, look for pathognomonic "saw-toothed pattern"

f. In patients with variable AV block or on AV node-blocking medications, the ventricular rate may be slower and irregular

4. Atrioventricular nodal reentrant tachycardia (AVNRT)

a. Caused by reentrant electrical loop involving the AV node and atrium, causing two conduits to form within the AV node: A slow conducting and a fast conducting

b. The slow pathway conducts both anterograde to the ventricle and retrograde toward the atrium near the tricuspid valve; this leads to simultaneous conduction of the both the atrium and ventricle

c. Therefore, P waves are rarely visualized in AVNRT, however, may be appreciated occasionally in the terminal aspect of QRS in lead V1

d. Heart rates typically range from 150 to 250 beats per minute with regular ventricular response, though typically 180–200 bpm

e. AHA/ACC: Often seen in young, healthy adults without structural heart disease

5. Atrioventricular reciprocating tachycardia (AVRT)

a. Caused by a bypass tract from the atrium to the ventricle within the cardiac musculature that extends beyond the tricuspid and mitral valves, which typically block any AV conduction; these bypass tracts can be anterograde, retrograde, or capable of both directions; pre-excitation refers to early activation of the ventricles due to impulses bypassing the AV node through this bypass tract

b. Heart rates typically range from 150 to 250 beats per minute with regular ventricular response

c. Delta wave: An initial upward slope of the QRS complex; present only in anterograde impulse, which signifies depolarization of ventricular tissue from conduction of the atrium to the ventricle along the bypass tract

   i. Delta waves are not visualized if there is no anterograde conduction

   ii. Delta wave + tachycardia: This signifies Wolf-Parkinson-White (WPW)

      iii. If delta wave without tachycardia, not WPW, but high risk for SVTs
         1. Short PR interval
         2. Delta wave
         3. Prolonged QRS >110 ms
   d. Orthodromic: Conduction through the AV node, with retrograde conduction back up through the bypass tract; narrow QRS with regular rhythm
   e. Antidromic: Anterograde conduction down bypass tract with retrograde conduction back up through the AV node; wide QRS with regular rhythm
   f. AF: Multiple atrial foci leading to extensive conduction along bypass tracts; wide QRS with irregular rhythm

6. Non-sinus focal atrial tachycardia
   a. Localized automatic focus within the atria, or small reentrant circuit within the atria
   b. P wave before every QRS, though different morphology compared to SA node
   c. Often occur in short, frequent bursts
   d. Atrial rate typically increases over initial 10 seconds of arrhythmia, then stabilizes to roughly 150–250 beats per minute
   e. Often seen in CAD, COPD, alcohol use
   f. AHA/ACC: Can distinguish sinus node reentry from sinus tachycardia by
      i. Abrupt onset and termination
      ii. Longer RP interval compared to normal sinus rhythm

7. MAT: Caused by multiple atrial foci with increased automaticity irritated by increased atrial pressures or hypoxia; often seen in COPD, pulmonary hypertension, coronary disease, valvular heart disease, hypomagnesemia, and theophylline therapy (AHA/ACC)
   a. Irregularly irregular rhythm with three or more distinct P wave morphologies before every QRS
   b. Heart rate typically between 100 and 150 beats per minute

8. AHA/ACC: Junctional tachycardia
   a. A rapid, narrow complex arrhythmia arising from the AV junction, including the bundle of His
   b. There are two types, junctional ectopic tachycardia (JET) and accelerated junctional rhythm (AJR)
      i. JET: Rare in adults, often seen in infants or after cardiac surgery in patients with CHF
         1. Typically a regular rhythm, though occasionally is irregular
         2. Narrow complex
         3. HR 120–220 bpm

    4. AV dissociation

    5. Due to focus within AV node; need to rate control if symptomatic

  ii. AJR: Occurs when AV node automaticity occurs at a rate faster than SA node or atrial foci

    1. Narrow complex, QRS <120 ms

    2. Retrograde P waves may be visible due to conduction into atria

    3. HR 70–130 bpm

    4. Often caused by digoxin toxicity; assess for upsloping ST segments throughout and assess digoxin levels; myocardial ischemia may also be a contributor, therefore, if any risk rule out ischemia

Acute Medical Management (AHA/ACC/HRS 2015)

1. Sinus tachycardia: Most often caused by underlying illness, anemia, hyperthyroid, etc.; treat underlying disease; if inappropriate sinus tachycardia (IST), and no underlying cause found after full workup, consider ivabradine

  a. Ivabradine is an inhibitor to I-funny channel which is responsible for normal automaticity of the sinus node

  b. Start 5 mg PO BID

  c. Limited to only SA node, therefore helpful only in IST, with no hemodynamic effects other than lowering HR

  d. Cardiovascular training may be of benefit, but no evidence has proven benefit

2. Non-sinus focal atrial tachycardia: No good trials or evidence to support treatment; may use vagal maneuvers to rule out other causes and distinguish this identity

  a. Beta blocker, diltiazem, or verapamil can decrease heart rate and is appropriate in hemodynamically stable patients

  b. Synchronized cardioversion for those who are hemodynamically unstable

  c. For ongoing management, catheter ablation or beta blockers/calcium channel blockers are appropriate management

3. MAT: Antiarrhythmic medications and cardioversion are typically not helpful in MAT

  a. Treat the underlying condition!

  b. Treat with metoprolol IV or verapamil IV for acute exacerbation

  c. For ongoing treatment, verapamil, diltiazem, or metoprolol orally is effective

4. AVNRT: Initially start with noninvasive maneuvers, then move to electrical cardioversion if necessary

  a. Vagal maneuvers

  b. Adenosine1 6 mg IV × 1, followed by 12 mg IV q1–2 min × 1–2 as needed

    c. Perform synchronized cardioversion for acute treatment in hemodynamically unstable patients with AVNRT when adenosine and vagal maneuvers do not terminate the tachycardia or are not feasible

    d. If patient refuses electrical cardioversion, can use beta blocker or CCB; if this fails to control heart rate, transition to flecainide or propafenone if no structural heart disease or use amiodarone if structural heart disease is present

5. Orthodromic AVRT: Accounts for 90%–95% of all accessory pathway SVTs

    a. Vagal maneuvers

    b. Adenosine 6 mg IV × 1, followed by 12 mg IV q1–2 min × 1–2 as needed

    c. Perform synchronized cardioversion for acute treatment in hemodynamically unstable patients with AVRT when adenosine and vagal maneuvers do not terminate the tachycardia or are not feasible

    d. Diltiazem, verapamil, and BBs safe in orthodromic AVRT if NO evidence of pre-excitation and inability to control with above therapies

    e. Offer catheter ablation for all AVRT; if patient refuses, or not a candidate, consider antiarrhythmics including propafenone, flecainide (if no structural disease), or amiodarone, sotalol, ibutilide

    f. Oral beta blockers, diltiazem, or verapamil are indicated for ongoing management of AVRT in patients without pre-excitation on their resting ECG

6. Pre-excited AVRT including antidromic AVRT: Typically wide-complex tachycardia secondary to pre-excitation along accessory pathway as noted above

    a. Avoid adenosine as this can precipitate AF, leading to increased conduction along accessory pathway and ultimately ventricular fibrillation

    b. Avoid verapamil, diltiazem, and BBs as it can lead to profound hypotension

    c. NEJM: Electrical cardioversion necessary for unstable wide-complex arrhythmias

    d. NEJM: Procainamide, ibutilide, amiodarone, propafenone are helpful in termination and can be used in pre-excitation pathways

    e. If a candidate, always offer catheter ablation of the accessory pathway

7. Atrial flutter: Treatment is very similar to AF, and also requires anticoagulation given increased stroke and thrombus risk

    a. Synchronized cardioversion for those who are hemodynamically unstable

    b. Dofetilide or ibutilide are effective for pharmacological cardioversion

    c. Beta blocker, diltiazem, or verapamil can decrease heart rate and is appropriate in hemodynamically stable patients

    d. For ongoing management, catheter ablation of the cavotricuspid isthmus; beta blockers/calcium channel blockers are appropriate management to control rate if hemodynamically stable

e. Acute and ongoing management require antithrombotic therapy, as per AF guidelines

8. Junctional tachycardia: Assess JET versus AJR

   a. Acute: Intravenous beta blockers are first line for symptomatic patients; IV diltiazem, procainamide, or verapamil are reasonable substitutes acutely

   b. Chronic: Oral beta blockers, verapamil, or diltiazem; catheter ablation may be necessary if refractory to all medication

Sources:

1. AHA/ACC/HRS 2015: Page RL, Joglar JA, Caldwell MA, et al. 2015 ACC/AHA/HRS guideline for the management of adult patients with supraventricular tachycardia. J Am Coll Cardiol. 2016;67(13):e27–e115. [https://www.ncbi.nlm.nih.gov/pubmed/26409259]

   a. Link, M. Evaluation and initial treatment of supraventricular tachycardia. NEJM. 2012;367(15):1438–1448. [https://www.ncbi.nlm .nih.gov/pubmed/23050527]

INFECTIVE ENDOCARDITIS

Initial Assessment (ACC/AHA/IDSA 2015, ESC 2015)

1. Blood cultures

   a. Obtain at least three sets of blood cultures from different venipuncture sites with first and last samples drawn at least 1 hour apart

   b. Repeat positive initial blood cultures

   c. ACC/AHA: Every 24–48 hours until bacteremia has cleared

   d. ESC: Once at 48–72 hours

   e. If all cultures negative, consider workup for noninfectious endocarditis

   f. ESC: Obtain three sets of blood cultures in patients with cardiac devices, including culturing from the lead-tip when device is explanted

2. Imaging

   a. Perform TTE within 12 hours or sooner for all cases of suspected IE

   b. If TTE is positive, perform TEE as soon as possible

   c. Repeat negative TEE

   d. ACC/AHA: In 3–5 days, if suspicion is high or clinical course worsening

   e. ESC: In 5–7 days

   f. ESC: Perform TEE in all patients with prosthetic valves or intracardiac devices

   g. ESC: Repeat TTE and/or TEE if new complication develops[17]

   h. ESC: Consider echocardiogram in all cases of staph bacteremia

---

[17]Complicated endocarditis: murmurs, valve dysfunction, embolism, persisting fever, HF, abscess, AV block.

  i. Consider additional imaging such as 3D ECHO, CT-angiogram, and MRI to assess for CNS and intra-abdominal lesions such as splenic infarctions[18]

Acute Medical Management (ACC/AHA/IDSA 2015, ESC 2015)

1. Choice of antibiotic
   a. See Table 1-3 for recommendations based on specific pathogens
   b. General principles: Choice of initial empiric therapy depends on
      i. Whether previous antibiotics received
      ii. Native valve or prosthetic valve and timing since surgery
      iii. Setting where infection was obtained (i.e., community or nosocomial)
2. Duration of antibiotics:
   a. ACC: Duration begins with the first day blood cultures are negative, if blood cultures are initially positive
   b. ESC: Prosthetic valve endocarditis (PVE): Treat with at least 6 weeks of antibiotics
   c. ESC: Native valve endocarditis (NVE): Treat with antibiotics for 2–6 weeks
   d. ESC: If initially NVE, but requires valve replacement during antibiotic treatment, then give postoperative antibiotic regimen for NVE not PVE
   e. ESC: Treat patients with intracardiac devices with prolonged course of antibiotic therapy

Interventions (ACC/AHA/IDSA 2015, ESC 2015)

1. Cardiac surgery: May be indicated in the following circumstances[19]
   a. Cardiac complications
      i. Heart failure, heart arrhythmia (i.e., heart block), hemodynamic instability
      ii. Annular or aortic abscess
      iii. Fistula or false aneurysm
      iv. Valve dysfunction or severe valve regurgitation
      v. Destructive, enlarging, or penetrating lesions
   b. Persistent infection
      i. Bacteremia or fever despite antibiotic treatment lasting >5–7 days
      ii. PVE caused by staphylococci or non-HACEK gram-negative bacteria
      iii. Fungal IE
   c. Prevention of pulmonary emboli
      i. Aortic or mitral NVE or PVE with persistent or enlarging vegetations despite appropriate antibiotic therapy

---

[18]Consider risks such as radiation exposure and nephrotoxicity.
[19]ACC/AHA: Avoid surgery when possible in patients who are intravenous drug users.

TABLE 1-3

CHOICE OF ANTIBIOTIC IN INFECTIVE ENDOCARDITIS

Bacterial Species	Native Valve	Prosthetic Valve	Comment
Empiric/Culture negative	ACC/AHA/IDSA 1. Acute IE: Vancomycin + cefepime 2. Subacute IE: Vancomycin + ampicillin/sulbactam ESC 1. Ampicillin + oxacillin + gentamicin 2. If PCN allergy, vancomycin + gentamicin	ACC/AHA/IDSA 1. <12 months post-surgery: Vancomycin + rifampin + gentamicin + cefepime 2. ≥12 months post-surgery: Vancomycin + ceftriaxone ESC 1. <12 months post-surgery: Vancomycin + rifampin + gentamicin 2. ≥12 months post-surgery: Vancomycin + gentamicin	• Consult infectious disease specialist early to guide antibiotic choices • If culture negative, consider ruling out anti-phospholipid antibody, fungal, or viral causes
Streptococcal: Bovis Viridans group	Ceftriaxone or PCN alone × 4 weeks[1] Ceftriaxone or PCN + gentamicin × 2 weeks	Ceftriaxone or PCN × 6 weeks May include gentamicin for first 2 weeks	If PCN resistant (MIC >0.12 μg/mL), add gentamicin
Streptococcal: *Abitropha defectiva* *Granulicatella* species Viridans group with MIC ≥0.5 μg/mL	Ampicillin or PCN + Gentamicin (ID consultation for duration) May use ceftriaxone instead of ampicillin/PCN if susceptible	ID consultation	

(Continued)

TABLE 1-3 *(Continued)*

CHOICE OF ANTIBIOTIC IN INFECTIVE ENDOCARDITIS

Bacterial Species	Native Valve	Prosthetic Valve	Comment
Streptococcal: Pneumoniae Pyogenes Groups B, C, F, G	PCN, cefazolin, or ceftriaxone × 4 weeks Consider adding gentamicin for first 2 weeks if group B, C, or G	PCN, cefazolin, or ceftriaxone × 6 weeks	IE from these organisms is rare; consult ID If PCN resistant *S. pneumoniae* **without** meningitis, use high doses of penicillin or 3rd generation cephalosporin If *S. pneumoniae* **with** meningitis, treat with cefotaxime instead
Staphylococcal Methicillin-sensitive *Staphylococcus aureus* (MSSA)	Right-sided valve (RV): Nafcillin × 2–4 weeks Left-sided valve: Nafcillin × 6 weeks Do not give gentamicin (aminoglycosides) or rifampin	Nafcillin + rifampin × 6 weeks + Gentamicin × 2 weeks	RV IE: If complicated (renal failure, metastatic pulmonary infection, MRSA, meningitis) extend duration to 6 weeks Per ESC: Treat with flucloxacillin or oxacillin 4–6 weeks or clotrimoxazole with clindamycin Use cefazolin instead of beta-lactams if patient has non-anaphylactoid reaction If brain abscess complicating MSSA IE, treat with nafcillin rather than cefazolin *Use daptomycin as an alternative to vancomycin*

Staphylococcal	Vancomycin × 6 weeks[2]	Vancomycin + rifampin × at least 6 weeks and gentamicin × 2 weeks	ESC: Give rifampin after 3–5 days of effective antibiotic therapy
Methicillin-resistant *Staphylococcus aureus* (MRSA)	Alternatively: Daptomycin × 6 weeks		If resistant to aminoglycosides, fluoroquinolones may be acceptable
Enterococci	Ampicillin or PCN + gentamicin Duration: 4 weeks if symptom duration <3 months[3] 6 weeks if symptom duration >3 months	Ampicillin or PCN + gentamicin × 6 weeks	If CrCl <50 mL/h use double beta lactam coverage × 6 weeks
Haemophilus Aggregatibacter Cardiobacterium Eikenella Kingella	Ceftriaxone (1st line) Alternates: Ciprofloxacin Duration: 4 weeks	Ceftriaxone (1st line) Alternates: Ciprofloxacin Duration: 4 weeks (ESC: 6 weeks)	
Fungal	Amphotericin for *Candida* Voriconazole for *Aspergillus* Duration: 6 weeks	Amphotericin for *Candida* Voriconazole for *Aspergillus* Duration: 6 weeks	Give life-long suppression with azole after therapy completed

[1] If intolerant to penicillin or ceftriaxone, may treat with 4 weeks of vancomycin monotherapy.
[2] Trough goal: 10–20 μg/mL.
[3] ESC: 4–6 weeks of amoxicillin + 2–4 weeks gentamicin.
Sources: ACC/AHA/IDSA 2015, ESC 2015.

ii. Isolated large vegetation >0.30 mm

iii. Recurrent emboli

iv. ESC: Silent embolism or TIA

v. Consider valve surgery for persisting vegetations in patients with stroke, subclinical cerebral emboli, if ICH excluded, and no severe neurological damage (i.e., coma)

vi. If major stroke of ICH, delay valve surgery for 4 weeks

d. ESC: Consider complete removal of infected devices

Management After Stabilization (ACC/AHA/IDSA 2015, ESC 2015)

1. Monitoring

a. Repeat TTE at completion of antibiotic therapy

2. Anticoagulation

a. ACC/AHA/IDSA 2015:

i. Stop all anticoagulation for at least 2 weeks in patients with mechanical valve IE with CNS embolic events

1. Reintroduce anticoagulation carefully with UFH to goal PTT 50–70s before oral warfarin

2. Do not use novel anticoagulants in valves with risks for embolism

ii. Do not start/initiate aspirin or antiplatelet agents as adjunctive therapy in IE, however, consider continuing aspirin/antiplatelet agents if there are no bleeding complications for patients already on those therapies

b. ESC 2015

i. Stop all anticoagulation in the presence of major bleeding, including ICH

ii. Avoid thrombolytic therapy

iii. If patient develops ischemic stroke without hemorrhage, replace oral anticoagulant therapy with unfractionated or low-molecular-weight heparin for 1–2 weeks

iv. If patient develops ICH with mechanical valve, reinitiate unfractionated or low-molecular-weight heparin as soon as possible (see section "Valvular Heart Disease" on anticoagulation below)

Sources:

1. ACC/AHA/IDSA 2015: Baddour LM, Wilson WR, Bayer AS, et al. Infective endocarditis in adults: diagnosis, antimicrobial therapy, and management of complications. Circulation. 2015;132(15):1435–1486. [https://www.ncbi.nlm.nih.gov/pubmed/26373316]

2. ESC 2015: Habib G, Lancellotti P, Antunes MJ, et al. 2015 ESC guidelines for the management of infective endocarditis. Eur Herat J. 2015;36(44):3075–3128. [https://www.ncbi.nlm.nih.gov/pubmed/26320109]

3. ACR Appropriateness 2014: Hsu JY, Malik SB, Abbara S, et al. ACR Appropriateness Criteria® suspected infective endocarditis [online publication]. Reston (VA): American College of Radiology (ACR); 2014. 8 p. [https://acsearch.acr.org/docs/69408/Narrative/]

VALVULAR HEART DISEASE

Initial Assessment (ACC/AHA 2014, ESC 2012)

1. Imaging
   a. Get echocardiogram for all cases of suspected valvular heart disease or known valvular disease with any change in symptoms
   b. Get coronary angiography
      i. ESC: Before valve surgery if patient has cardiac risk factors
      ii. ACC/AHA: If valve imaging inconclusive, or if patient symptomatic with a physical exam suggestive of severe lesion
   c. Get exercise testing
      i. ACC/AHA: In patients with asymptomatic severe VHD[20] to confirm absence of symptoms, assess hemodynamic response to exercise, or determine prognosis
2. Consulting: Consult cardiology/cardiothoracic surgery for severe valvular disease (see below)

Acute Medical Management (ACC/AHA 2014)

1. Aortic stenosis (AS)
   a. Treat hypertension with goal-directed medial therapy (GDMT) in at-risk patients who are asymptomatic
   b. For decompensated AS, use vasodilator therapy with increased monitoring (usually ICU)
   c. Do not use statin therapy to prevent AS in patients with mild-to-moderate disease
2. Aortic regurgitation (AR)
   a. Treat hypertension with dihydropyridine CCB and ACEi/ARBS
   b. If severe AR with LV dysfunction and surgery is not performed, give ACEi/ARBs and beta blocker
3. Mitral stenosis (MS)
   a. Anticoagulate patients with MS and AF, previous embolic event of left atrial thrombus (see section "Atrial Fibrillation")
   b. Control heart rate
   c. Secondary prevention of rheumatic fever is indicated in patients with rheumatic heart disease
4. Mitral regurgitation (MR)
   a. Treat systolic dysfunction in chronic MR, if surgery is not being considered
   b. If chronic primary MR and normotensive, do not use vasodilator therapy
   c. If chronic secondary MR with heart failure (HF), use GDMT and consider CRT with biventricular pacing

---

[20]Exception: Do not perform exercise stress testing for patients with severe aortic stenosis.

5. Tricuspid regurgitation (TR)
   a. In severe TR with signs of right HF, consider diuretics and medical therapy to reduce pulmonary artery pressures

Interventions (ACC/AHA 2014)

See Table 1-4 for indications for valvular surgery

Management After Stabilization (ACCP 2012)

1. Antithrombotic therapy after valve replacement/repair
   a. Mechanical valves
      i. Aortic: VKA therapy, target INR range 2.0–3.0
      ii. Mitral: VKA therapy, target INR range 2.5–3.5

TABLE 1-4

INDICATIONS FOR SURGICAL VALVE REPAIR (VR)/TRANSCATHETER VALVE REPLACEMENT (TVR)/PERCUTANEOUS BALLOON DILATION		
Valve Disorder	**Threshold for Surgical Consult**	**Comment**
Aortic regurgitation	Severe valve disease AND one of the following: • Symptoms • LVEF <50%[1]	
Aortic stenosis	Severe high-gradient AS AND one of the following: • Symptoms (history or on stress test) • Asymptomatic with LVEF <50% (Stage C2 or worse)[2] • Undergoing cardiac surgery for other indication	Aortic valve area <1 cm^2 indicates poor prognosis
Mitral stenosis	Severe MS (Stage D, valve area ≤1.5 cm^2) AND one of the following: • Symptoms,[3] but without LA thrombus or moderate-to-severe MR (percutaneous mitral balloon commissurotomy is preferred over valve surgery) • Severe symptoms (NYHA class III/IV) • Cardiac surgery for other indication	May see severe LA enlargement and pulmonary systolic arterial pressure (PASP) >30 mmHg ECC 2012: Consider intervention in asymptomatic patients with preserved LV function who develop AF or pulmonary hypertension

(Continued)

TABLE 1-4 (*Continued*)

INDICATIONS FOR SURGICAL VALVE REPAIR (VR)/TRANSCATHETER VALVE REPLACEMENT (TVR)/PERCUTANEOUS BALLOON DILATION

Valve Disorder	Threshold for Surgical Consult	Comment
Mitral regurgitation (MR)	Acute severe primary[4] MR	Mitral valve repair is preferred over replacement when valve morphology allows and skilled practitioner available
	Chronic severe primary MR (Stage D) AND one of the following:	
	• Symptoms with LVEF >30%[5]	
	• Asymptomatic with LVEF 30%–60%	
	• Cardiac surgery for other indication	
Tricuspid regurgitation	Severe TR, when undergoing mitral or aortic valve surgery	
	Mild/moderate TR, when undergoing mitral or aortic valve surgery, if tricuspid annular dilation or prior evidence of HF	
Tricuspid stenosis	Severe TS, when undergoing mitral or aortic valve surgery	
	Isolated, symptomatic, severe TS	
Prosthetic valve thrombosis	Left-sided valve thrombosis, NYHA class III/IV symptoms[6]	
	AND/OR	
	Mobile, large thrombus (>0.8 cm^2)	
Prosthetic valve stenosis	Severe, symptomatic stenosis	
Prosthetic valve regurgitation	Mechanical valve AND intractable hemolysis or HF due to regurgitation	

[1]Weaker recommendation for considering surgery if EF >50% but severe LV dilation.
[2]Weaker recommendation for considering surgery if Stage C1, aortic velocity >5.0 m/s, and surgical risk low.
[3]Weaker recommendation for considering surgery in asymptomatic patients with very severe MS (valve area ≤1.0 cm^2, Stage C) who are favorable surgical candidates.
[4]Primary MR refers to a mechanical failure of a component of the valve (leaflets, chordae tendinae, papillary muscles, annulus). Secondary MR refers to a normal valve that is compromised by severe LV dysfunction.
[5]Weaker recommendation exists for surgery patients with LVEF <30% – the benefit/risk ratio is less pronounced.
[6]Weaker recommendation for consideration of surgery in mobile or large thrombus (>8 mm), regardless of symptoms.
Source: Adapted from ACC/AHA 2014.

        iii. Bridge with UFH or LMWH until stable on VKA

        iv. If low bleeding risk, add aspirin 81 mg to VKA therapy

        v. Do not use oral direct thrombin inhibitors or anti-Xa agents in place of VKA

    b. Bioprosthetic valves

        i. Aortic, sinus rhythm: Give aspirin 81 mg for 3 months, rather than VKA therapy

        ii. Aortic, transcatheter: Give aspirin 81 mg and clopidogrel 75 mg for 3 months, rather than VKA therapy

        iii. Mitral: Give VKA therapy, target INR range 2.0–3.0, for 3 months

2. Peri-procedural anticoagulation for prosthetic valves

    a. Minor procedures (i.e., dental extractions, cataract removal): Continue anticoagulation at goal therapeutic INR

    b. Invasive surgical procedures, bileaflet mechanical aortic valve but low risk for thrombosis: Temporarily stop VKA anticoagulation, without bridging

    c. Invasive surgical procedures, other mechanical valves: Bridge anticoagulation with UFH or subcutaneous low-molecular-weight heparin (LMWH) while INR subtherapeutic

Sources:

1. ACC/AHA 2014: Nishimura, RA, Otto, CM, Bonow, RO, et al. 2014 AHA/ACC guideline for the management of patients with valvular heart disease. Circulation. 2014;123(23):2440–2492. [https://www.ncbi.nlm.nih.gov/pubmed/24589852]

2. ESC 2012: Joint task force on the management of valvular heart disease of the European Society of Cardiology. Guidelines on the management of valvular heart disease (version 2012). Eur Heart J. 2012;33(19):2451–2496. [https://www.ncbi.nlm.nih.gov/pubmed/22922415]

3. ACCP 2012: Whitlock, RP, Sun, JC, Fremes, SE, et al. Antithrombotic and thrombolytic therapy for valvular disease: antithrombotic therapy and prevention of thrombosis, 9th ed: American College of Chest Physicians evidence-based clinical practice guidelines. Chest. 2012;141(2 Suppl):e576S–e600S. [http://www.guideline.gov/content.aspx?id=35271]

Vascular

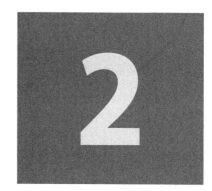

Zachary Zwolak
James Rohlfing

VENOUS THROMBOEMBOLISM

Initial Assessment

1. Deep venous thrombosis (ACCP 2012)
   a. For suspected initial DVT, use Wells score for DVT to determine pretest probability and therefore diagnostic algorithm[1]
      i. Wells score for DVT (NEJM. 349(13))
         1. Assign one point for each of the following
            a. Active cancer
            b. Immobility of lower extremities
            c. Bedridden 3+ days in past 3 months
            d. Tenderness along deep vein
            e. Swollen leg
            f. Unilateral calf swelling (3 cm larger than other)
            g. Unilateral pitting edema
            h. Collateral venous distention
            i. History of prior DVT
         2. Remove 2 points if an alternate diagnosis is as likely as DVT
   b. Diagnostic algorithms
      i. Low pretest probability, lower extremity DVT: See Figure 2-1
      ii. Moderate pretest probability, lower extremity DVT: See Figure 2-2
      iii. High pretest probability, lower extremity DVT: See Figure 2-3
      iv. Suspicion of recurrent lower extremity DVT: See Figure 2-4
2. Pulmonary embolism (ACCP 2016)

---

[1]Wells score was validated in the outpatient setting and may not perform as well in the inpatient setting. Do not allow a low Wells score to override your clinical suspicion of VTE (JAMA Intern Med. 2015;175(7)).

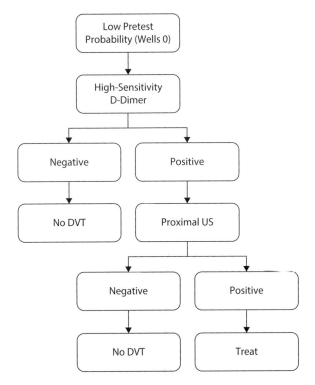

FIGURE 2-1. Diagnostic algorithm for suspected low pretest probability initial lower extremity DVT. (Adapted from ACCP 2012.)

a. For suspected pulmonary embolism, use Wells score for PE or revised Geneva score for PE, creatinine clearance, and age-adjusted D-dimer to guide diagnostic strategy
 i. Revised Geneva score for PE (Ann Intern Med. 144(3))
  1. Assign points for HR
   a. 5 points if ≥95
   b. 3 points if 75–94
  2. Assign 4 points for: Tender lower extremity
  3. Assign 3 points for each of
   a. History of DVT/PE
   b. Painful lower extremity
  4. Assign 2 points for each of
   a. Surgery or fractured lower extremity (in past month)
   b. Active malignancy (in past year)
   c. Hemoptysis
  5. Assign 1 point for age >65
b. For diagnostic algorithm, see Figure 2-5

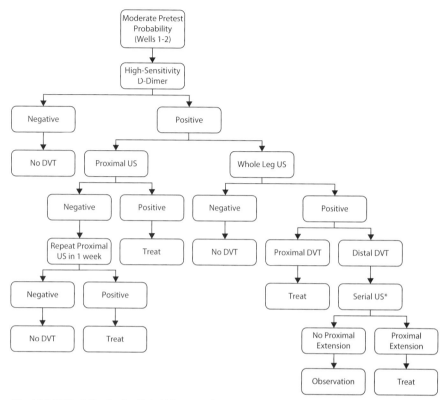

* Treat distal DVT only if patient is at high-risk for proximal extension or severely symptomatic.

FIGURE 2-2. Diagnostic algorithm for suspected moderate pretest probability initial lower extremity DVT. (Adapted from ACCP 2012.)

Acute Medical Management (ACCP 2012, 2016)

1. Anticoagulation: Decision to anticoagulate, anticoagulant selection, and duration of therapy guided by multiple factors
2. For DVT: See Table 2-1 for anticoagulant selection
3. For PE, see Figure 2-6 for treatment algorithm and Table 2-2 for anticoagulant selection

Management After Stabilization (ACCP 2016)

1. If low-risk PE and home circumstances are adequate, treat at home or discharge early rather than the standard discharge after 5 days of treatment

Sources:

1. ACCP 2012: Bates SM, Jaeschke R, Stevens SM, et al. Antithrombotic therapy and prevention of thrombosis, 9th ed: American College of Chest Physicians evidence-based clinical practice guidelines. Chest. February 2012;131(2): 351–418. [https://www.ncbi.nlm.nih.gov/pmc/articles/PMC3278048/]

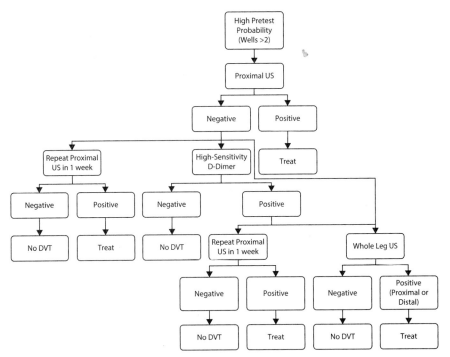

In patients with extensive unexplained leg swelling, if there is no DVT on proximal CUS or whole-leg US and D-dimer testing has not been performed or is positive, the iliac veins should be imaged to exclude isolated iliac DVT.

FIGURE 2-3. Diagnostic algorithm for suspected high pretest probability initial lower extremity DVT. (Adapted from ACCP 2012.)

2. ACCP 2015: Kearon C, Akl EA, Omelas J, et al. Antithrombotic therapy for VTE disease. CHEST Guideline and Expert Panel Report. Chest. 2016;149(2):315–352. [https://www.ncbi.nlm.nih.gov/pubmed/26867832]

3. ACP 2015: Raja AS, Greenberg JO, Qaseem A, et al. Evaluation of patients with suspected acute pulmonary embolism: best practice advice from the Clinical Guidelines Committee of the American College of Physicians. Ann Intern Med. 2015;163:701–711. [https://www.ncbi.nlm.nih.gov/pubmed/26414967]

4. Wells PS, Anderson DR, Rodger M, et al. Evaluation of D-dimer in the diagnosis of suspected deep-venous thrombosis. NEJM. 2003;394(13):1227–1235. [https://www.ncbi.nlm.nih.gov/pubmed/14507948]

5. Silveira PC, Ip IK, Goldhaber SZ, et al. Performance of Wells score for deep vein thrombosis in the inpatient setting. JAMA Intern Med. 2015;175(7):1112–1117. [https://www.ncbi.nlm.nih.gov/pubmed/25985219]

6. Le Gal G, Righini M, Roy PM, et al. Prediction of pulmonary embolism in the emergency department: the revised Geneva score. Ann Intern Med. 2006;144(3):165–171. [https://www.ncbi.nlm.nih.gov/pubmed/16461960]

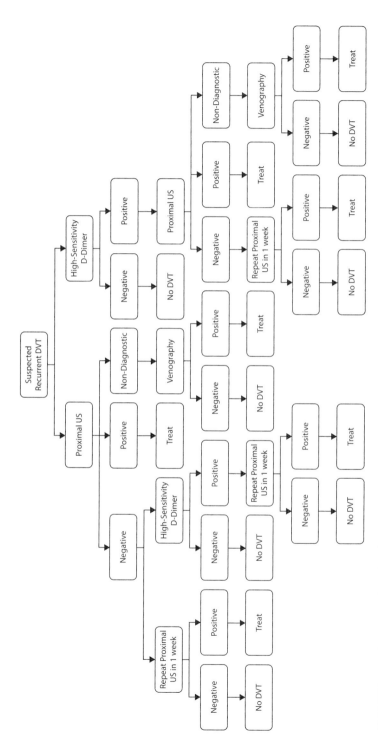

FIGURE 2-4. Diagnostic algorithm for suspected recurrent lower extremity DVT. (Adapted from ACCP 2012.)

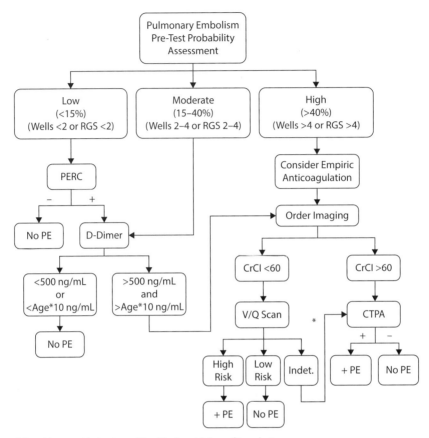

FIGURE 2-5. Diagnostic algorithm for suspected pulmonary embolism. (Adapted from ACCP 2012.)

PERIPHERAL ARTERIAL DISEASE

Initial Assessment (ACCF/AHA 2011)

1. Ankle brachial index (ABI), toe brachial index, and segmental pressure examination
   a. Use ABI for diagnosis, not screening
   b. Diagnose PAD with ABI if patient has one or more of the following: Exertional leg symptoms, nonhealing wounds, age >65, age >50 with history of diabetes or smoking
   c. Measure ABI in both legs to establish a baseline and confirm diagnosis
   d. If ABI not reliable because of noncompressible vessels, use toe brachial index
   e. Use leg segmental pressures to anatomically localize PAD

f. ABI report: Noncompressible (>1.40), normal (1.00–1.40), borderline (0.91–0.99), and abnormal (<0.90)

Acute Medical Management

1. Acute limb ischemia (ACCP 2012)
   a. Use systemic anticoagulation with unfractionated heparin followed by reperfusion therapy
2. Critical limb ischemia (ACCP 2012)
   a. Consider vascular intervention
   b. If not candidate for vascular intervention, give prostanoids (alprostadil, ecraprost, epoprostenol) in addition to antithrombotics (aspirin or clopidogrel)
3. Tobacco cessation (ACCF/AHA 2011)
   a. Ask about smoking status at every encounter
   b. Advise to quit, assist with counseling, offer interventions, develop plan: Refer to cessation program or initiate pharmacotherapy
   c. In absence of contraindication, offer patients pharmacotherapy: Varenicline, bupropion, and nicotine replacement therapy[2]

Interventions

1. Reperfusion therapy (ACCP 2012)
   a. Surgery is preferred over interarterial (IA) thrombolysis
   b. IA thrombolysis with recombinant tissue-type plasminogen activator (rt-PA) or urokinase is preferred over streptokinase
2. Surgery for critical limb ischemia (ACCF/AHA 2011)
   a. If autologous vein conduit not available and life expectancy ≤2 years, then balloon angioplasty may be the initial procedure
   b. If autologous vein conduit available and life expectancy ≥2 years, then bypass surgery may be the initial procedure
3. Abdominal aortic aneurysm (AAA) surgery (ACCF/AHA 2011)
   a. Open or endovascular repair (EVAR) of infrarenal AAA ± iliac aneurysm is indicated in "good surgical candidates"[3]
   b. Open repair is preferred for patients who cannot comply with periodic surveillance required post-EVAR
   c. After AAA repair, monitor for endoleak, graft position, stability of aneurysm sac, and need for further intervention
4. Atherosclerotic renovascular disease: Benefit < risk for revascularization (ACCF/AHA 2011)

Management After Stabilization

1. Percutaneous transluminal angioplasty (with or without stenting): Give long-term aspirin or clopidogrel (but not dual antiplatelet therapy (DAPT)) (ACCP 2012)

---

[2]Success at 6 months verbal advice versus pharmacotherapy, 6.8% versus 21.3%. Success rates: Nicotine replacement, 16%; bupropion, 30%.
[3]"Good surgical candidate" is not defined in the guideline.

TABLE 2-1

RECOMMENDED ANTICOAGULANT SELECTION AND DURATION OF ANTICOAGULATION BASED ON RISK FACTORS AND LOCATION OF DVT

Limb	Prox vs. Dist	Provoked	Cancer	Bleeding Risk	Anticoagulants	Duration
Upper	Prox	Yes	Yes		No specific recommendations	Indefinite
			No		No specific recommendations	3 months
		No	No	High	No specific recommendations	3 months
				Low	No specific recommendations	Indefinite
	Dist[1]	Yes	Yes		No specific recommendations	Indefinite
			No		No specific recommendations	3 months
		No	No	High	No specific recommendations	3 months
				Low	No specific recommendations	Indefinite
Lower	Prox	Yes	Yes		LMWH over VKA, direct thrombin, or Xa inhibitors	Indefinite
			No		Dabigatran, rivaroxaban, apixaban, or edoxaban over VKA	3 months

			Treatment	Duration
No	No	High	Dabigatran, rivaroxaban, apixaban, or edoxaban over VKA	3 months
		Low	Dabigatran, rivaroxaban, apixaban, or edoxaban over VKA	Indefinite
Dist[1]	Yes	Yes	LMWH over VKA, direct thrombin, or Xa inhibitors	Indefinite
	No	No	Dabigatran, rivaroxaban, apixaban, or edoxaban over VKA	3 months
	No	High	Dabigatran, rivaroxaban, apixaban, or edoxaban over VKA	3 months
		Low	Dabigatran, rivaroxaban, apixaban, or edoxaban over VKA	Indefinite

[1]In general, treatment of isolated distal upper or lower extremity DVT is not recommended unless there are severe symptoms or a high risk for or evidence of proximal extension on ultrasound.

VKA, vitamin K antagonist.

Source: Adapted from ACCP 2016.

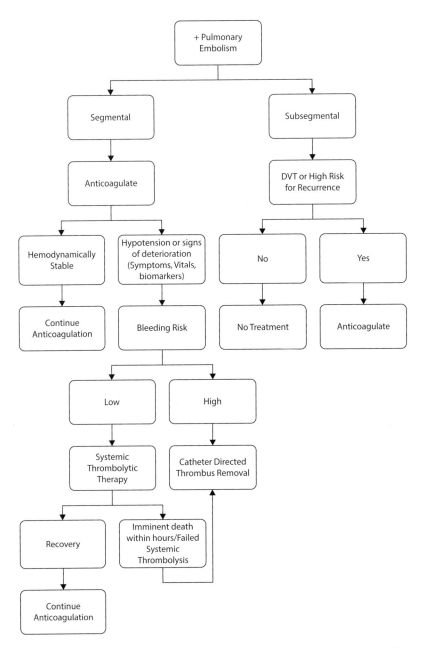

FIGURE 2-6. Treatment algorithm for confirmed pulmonary embolism. (Adapted from ACCP 2016.)

TABLE 2-2

RECOMMENDED ANTICOAGULANT SELECTION AND DURATION OF ANTICOAGULATION FOR PULMONARY EMBOLISM BASED ON RISK FACTORS AND LOCATION OF PULMONARY EMBOLISM

Location	Provoked	Cancer	Bleeding Risk	Anticoagulants	Duration
Segmental	Yes	Yes		LMWH over VKA, direct thrombin, or Xa inhibitors	Indefinite
	No	No		Dabigatran, rivaroxaban, apixaban, or edoxaban over VKA	3 months
		No	High	Dabigatran, rivaroxaban, apixaban, or edoxaban over VKA	3 months
			Low	Dabigatran, rivaroxaban, apixaban, or edoxaban over VKA therapy	Indefinite
Subsegmental[1]	Yes	Yes		LMWH over VKA, direct thrombin, or Xa inhibitors	Indefinite
		No		Dabigatran, rivaroxaban, apixaban, or edoxaban over VKA	3 months
	No	No	High	Dabigatran, rivaroxaban, apixaban, or edoxaban over VKA	3 months
			Low	Dabigatran, rivaroxaban, apixaban, or edoxaban over VKA	Indefinite

[1]In general, treatment of a subsegmental PE is not recommended unless there is a concomitant DVT or high risk for recurrence.
VKA, vitamin K antagonist.
Source: Adapted from ACCP 2016.

2. Peripheral artery bypass graft: Give aspirin 75–100 mg daily or clopidogrel 75 mg daily (ACCP 2012)

   a. Single agent preferred over warfarin and DAPT

   b. Below knee bypass graft with prosthetic graft: Clopidogrel 75 mg/day plus aspirin 75 mg for 1 year

   c. All other surgeries: Single antiplatelet agent preferred

3. Asymptomatic PAD (ACCP 2012, ACCF/AHA 2011)

   a. Give aspirin 75–100 mg if risk of MI is greater than risk of GI bleed for primary prevention of cardiovascular events

   b. ACCF/AHA: If ABI ≤0.90, give antiplatelet therapy; if ABI 0.91–0.99, benefit for antiplatelet therapy is not established

4. Symptomatic PAD (ACCP 2012, ACCF/AHA 2011)

   a. Symptoms: Intermittent claudication, limb ischemia, prior to revascularization and amputation

   b. Give aspirin for secondary prevention of MI, stroke, and vascular death

      i. ACCP: 75–100 mg daily

      ii. ACCF/AHA: 75–325 mg daily

   c. Clopidogrel: 75 mg daily, if patient cannot tolerate aspirin

   d. DAPT

      i. ACCP 2012: Do not use DAPT

      ii. ACCF/AHA: DAPT could be considered if bleeding risk is low and have a high perceived cardiovascular risk

   e. Warfarin: Do not use antiplatelet with moderate intensity warfarin[4]

Sources:

1. Rooke T, et al. 2011 ACCF/AHA focused update of the guideline for the management of patients with peripheral arterial disease (updating the 2005 guideline). Circulation. 2011;124:2020–2045. [https://www.ncbi.nlm.nih.gov/pubmed/22128043]

2. Alonso-Coello P, et al. Antithrombotic therapy and peripheral arterial disease: antithrombotic therapy and prevention of thrombosis, by physician: American College of Chest Physicians evidence-based guidelines. Chest. 2012:141(2):e669s–e690s. [http://journal.publications.chestnet.org/article.aspx?articleid=1159568]

---

[4] ACCF/AHA: Avoid warfarin in general while on antiplatelet therapy unless there is an alternate indication.

Pulmonary

3

Zachary Zwolak
James Rohlfing

PNEUMONIA

Initial Assessment
1. Determine disposition using illness severity score (NICE 2014)
   a. Assess severity: CRB 65 scale (see Table 3-1)
      i. 0: Low risk; <1% mortality
      ii. 1–2: Intermediate risk; 1%–10% mortality
      iii. 3–4: High risk; >10% mortality
   b. Disposition based on CRB 65 score
      i. 0–1: Care at home
      ii. ≥2: Hospital assessment
      iii. ≥3: ICU evaluation
2. Hospital admission determination (IDSA 2007)
   a. Use CURB 65 (CRB 65 plus uremia) to determine need for admission
   b. Use PSI/PORT score to determine severity
   c. Severe CAP if one major or three minor criteria
      i. Major
         1. Invasive mechanical ventilation
         2. Septic shock with need for vasopressors
      ii. Minor
         1. RR >30
         2. PaO_2/FiO_2 ratio ≤250
         3. Multilobular infiltrates
         4. Confusion/disorientation
         5. Uremia (BUN >20 mg/dL)
         6. Leukopenia (WBC <4000)
         7. Thrombocytopenia (platelet <100,000)
         8. Hypothermia (Temp <36°C)
         9. Hypotension requiring aggressive fluid resuscitation

TABLE 3-1

CRB 65 SCALE		
	Criteria	**Score**
C	Confusion (MMSE ≤8) or new delirium	1
R	Respiratory rate ≥30/min	1
B	BP ≤either SBP 90 mmHg or DBP 60 mmHg	1
65	Age ≥65 years	1

Source: Adapted from Thorax. 2003 May;58(5):377–382.

    d. ICU admission if
        i. Severe CAP
        ii. Septic shock requiring vasopressors
        iii. Acute respiratory failure requiring intubation and mechanical ventilation
    e. Laboratory testing (NICE 2014)
        i. CBC, CMP, lactate, HIV (if not tested recently)
        ii. CXR, 2-view
        iii. ABG if severe symptoms
        iv. CRP initially and repeat at 48–72 hours; if clinically indicated:
            1. Do not routinely offer antibiotic therapy if the CRP <20 mg/L
            2. Delay antibiotic prescription if CRP 20–100 mg/L
            3. Use antibiotic if CRP >100 mg/L
        v. Microbiological testing
            1. Obtain testing within 4 hours of presentation
            2. Low severity community-acquired pneumonia (CAP): No routine microbiological tests
            3. Moderate to high severity CAP: Obtain blood and sputum cultures, consider pneumococcal and *Legionella* urinary antigen test prior to antibiotic administration
            4. For testing based on risk factors, see Table 3-2
    f. Evaluation of suspected HAP/VAP (IDSA 2016)
        i. Cultures
            1. Noninvasive sampling with semiquantitative cultures is adequate; do not perform invasive sampling (i.e., BAL)
            2. If invasive means performed, but specimen below diagnostic threshold for VAP, consider withholding antibiotics
            3. Treatment based on results of noninvasive samples and deescalate antibiotic therapy based upon respiratory and blood culture results

TABLE 3-2

MICROBIOLOGICAL TESTING BASED ON PNEUMONIA RISK FACTORS

Indication	Blood Culture	Sputum Culture	Legionella UAT	Pneumococcal UAT	Other
Intensive care unit admission	X	X	X	X	X[1]
Failure of outpatient antibiotic therapy	X	X	X	X	
Cavitary infiltrates	X	X			X[2]
Leukopenia	X			X	
Active alcohol abuse	X	X	X	X	
Chronic severe liver disease	X			X	
Severe obstructive/structural lung disease		X			
Asplenia (anatomic or functional)	X				
Recent travel (within past 2 weeks)		X[4]	X		X[3]
Positive Legionella UAT result			NA		
Positive pneumococcal UAT result	X	X		NA	
Pleural effusion	X	X	X	X	X[5]

[1]Endotracheal aspirate if intubated, possibly bronchoscopy or nonbronchoscopic bronchoalveolar lavage.
[2]Fungal and tuberculosis cultures.
[3]See Table 8 in Mandell L, et al. Clin Infect Dis. 2007;S27–72 for details.
[4]Special media for *Legionella*.
[5]Thoracentesis and pleural fluid cultures.
Note: NA, not applicable; UAT, urinary antigen test.
Source: From IDSA 2007: Mandell L, et al. Infectious Diseases Society of America/American Thoracic Society consensus guidelines on the management of community-acquired pneumonia in adults. Clin Infect Dis. 2007;S27–S72 [https://www.ncbi.nlm.nih.gov/pubmed/17278083].

ii. Procalcitonin, C-reactive protein, sTREM-1 (soluble triggering receptor expressed on myeloid cells): Use clinical criteria alone rather than using these lab markers to decide to initiate antibiotics

Acute Medical Management

1. NICE: Initiate antibiotic therapy within 4 hours of admission
2. CAP
   a. Antibiotic therapy
      i. Low severity CAP, outpatient management
         1. Choice of antibiotic
            a. NICE 2016
               i. Give amoxicillin rather than macrolide or tetracycline for low severity CAP
               ii. Give macrolide or tetracycline if penicillin allergic
            b. IDSA 2007
               i. Do not routinely offer fluoroquinolone or dual antibiotic therapy (IDSA 2007)
               ii. If healthy and no risk for resistant *S. pneumoniae*: Macrolide (preferred) or doxycycline
               iii. If comorbidities are present (chronic heart, lung, liver, renal disease; diabetes; alcoholism; malignancy; asplenia, immunosuppression; recent antimicrobials within past 3 months), give:
                  1. Respiratory fluoroquinolone
                  2. Beta-lactam (amoxicillin 1 g TID or Amox-clav 2 g BID, or ceftriaxone, cefpodoxime, cefuroxime) + (macrolide (preferred) or doxycycline)
         2. Duration (NICE 2016)
            a. 5-day course of single antibiotic
            b. Extend course >5 days for low severity CAP with symptoms not improving after 3 days
   3. Moderate and high severity CAP
      a. Choice of antibiotic
         i. NICE
            1. Dual therapy with amoxicillin and macrolide
            2. Dual antibiotic with beta-lactamase and macrolide for high severity CAP
      b. Duration
         i. NICE: 7–10 day course
         ii. IDSA: Minimum of 5 days and afebrile >48–72 hours
         iii. Longer course if extrapulmonary infection, necrotizing PNA, empyema, or lung abscess

      iv. If no response to initial therapy >72 hours, consider resistance, superinfection, complication, delayed host response, incorrect diagnosis, metastatic infectious focus

  c. ICU treatment – Choice of antibiotic (IDSA 2007)

      i. Beta-lactam (cefotaxime, ceftriaxone, ampicillin/sulbactam) + (azithromycin or doxycycline or fluoroquinolone)

      ii. PCN allergy: Respiratory fluoroquinolone and aztreonam

      iii. *Pseudomonas* infection: Anti-pneumococcal + anti-pseudomonal regimen

        1. Anti-pneumococcal, anti-pseudomonal beta lactam + ciprofloxacin or levofloxacin (750 mg)

        2. Beta-lactam + aminoglycoside + azithromycin

        3. Beta-lactam + aminoglycoside + anti-pneumococcal fluoroquinolone

        4. PCN allergy: Aztreonam in place of beta-lactam

      iv. Community-acquired MRSA: Add vancomycin or linezolid

4. Influenza A (IDSA 2007)

  a. Give oseltamivir or zanamivir within 48 hours of symptom onset

      i. Do not give for uncomplicated influenza with symptoms >48 hours

      ii. May give after 48 hours of onset of symptoms for hospitalized patients to reduce viral shedding

5. Hospital-acquired pneumonia (HAP)

  a. Antibiotic therapy (NICE 2016, IDSA 2016 HAP/VAP)

      i. Initiate as soon as possible and within 4 hours

      ii. Duration of therapy

        1. IDSA: 7 days

        2. NICE: 5–10 days

      iii. Procalcitonin: Use with clinical criteria to discontinue therapy (see Table 3-3)

      iv. Choice of antibiotic

        1. Apply a local antibiogram

        2. IDSA: Empiric therapy: (pip-tazo, cefepime, levofloxacin, imipenem, or meropenem) + vancomycin or linezolid if MRSA risk

        3. *Pseudomonas aeruginosa*[1]: If non-septic, then use single agent; if septic, use dual anti-pseudomonal agents

        4. ESBL: Choose antibiotic based on susceptibility

        5. Acinetobacter: Carbapenem or ampicillin/sulbactam if susceptible

        6. Carbapenem-resistant organism: Polymyxins (colistin or polymyxin B)

---

[1] Risk for MDR or MRSA or MDR Pseudomonas HAP (IDSA 2016 HAP/VAP): If there has been IV antibiotic use within 90 days.

TABLE 3-3

USE OF PROCALCITONIN

1. Used to differentiate viral versus bacterial respiratory infection and guide antibiotic treatment length.
2. Not influenced by neutropenia.
3. If clinical condition is unstable, use clinical judgment over PCT level.
4. Follow PCT level every 24–48 hours as clinically indicated.

Non-pulmonary upper and/or lower respiratory tract infection in primary care or ED

PCT	≤0.1	<0.25	≥0.25	>0.5
Antibiotics	Strongly discouraged	Discouraged	Encouraged	Strongly encouraged

Pulmonary infections in hospital and ED settings

PCT result	≤0.1	<0.25	≥0.25	>0.5
Antibiotics	Strongly discouraged	Discouraged	Encouraged	Strongly encouraged

Sepsis and intubation and intensive care unit settings

PCT result	≤0.25	<0.5	≥0.5	>1
Antibiotics	Strongly discouraged	Discouraged	Encouraged	Strongly encouraged

Evaluation of cessation of antibiotics based on PCT level in septic patient

PCT result	≤0.25 or drop >90%	<0.5 or drop >80%	≥0.5	>1
Antibiotics cessation	Strongly discouraged	Discouraged	Encouraged	Strongly encouraged

Source: Adapted from Schuetz P, Amin DN, Greenwald JL. Role of procalcitonin in managing adult patients with respiratory tract infections. Chest. 2012 Apr;141(4):1063–1073.

    b. Ventilator-associated pneumonia (IDSA 2016 HAP/VAP)
       i. 7-day course preferred
      ii. Always attempt de-escalation
     iii. Procalcitonin: Use PCT + clinical criteria to discontinue therapy (Table 3-3)
        1. Risk for MDR VAP
          a. Prior IV antibiotics within 90 days (increases MRSA risk and MRD *Pseudomonas*)
          b. Septic shock at time of VAP
          c. ARDS preceding VAP

      d. ≥5 days of hospitalization prior to VAP

      e. Acute renal replacement therapy prior to VAP

  2. Choose antibiotics based on local antibiograms

  3. Pathogens: *S. aureus, P. aeruginosa*, and other gram-negative bacilli

      a. Treat for MRSA only if risk for resistance or >10%–20% of *S. aureus* isolates are MRSA

      b. Cover for MSSA only if low risk

      c. Cover with vancomycin or linezolid if MRSA coverage indicated, as opposed to other anti-MRSA agents

  4. MSSA: Pip-tazo, cefepime, levofloxacin, imipenem, or meropenem

  5. Antipseudomonal treatment

      a. Treat with dual antipseudomonal antibiotics if risk for resistance or >10% of gram-negative isolates in local setting are resistant

      b. If criteria not met, then single agent indicated

      c. If non-septic, then use single agent; if septic, use dual agents

  6. ESBL: Choose antibiotic based on susceptibility

  7. Acinetobacter: Carbapenem or ampicillin/sulbactam if susceptible

  8. Carbapenem resistant: Polymyxins (colistin or polymyxin B)

  9. Reserve use of aminoglycosides and colistin if other agents are available

Management After Stabilization

1. Discharge criteria (NICE 2016)

  a. Do not discharge if in past 24 hours, two or more of the following persist:

      i. Temp >37.5°C

      ii. RR >24

      iii. HR >100

      iv. SBP ≤90 mmHg

      v. SaO_2 <90% on RA

      vi. Abnormal mentation

      vii. Inability to eat without assistance

2. Vaccines and follow-up (IDSA 2007)

  a. Facilitate smoking cessation

  b. Influenza vaccine for all patients during fall and winter

  c. Pneumococcal polysaccharide vaccine for patients ≥65 years old and those with high-risk comorbidities

  d. Smokers who do not intend to quit: Influenza and pneumococcus vaccines

  e. Report cases of pneumonia that are a public health concern to state or local health department

Bonus Section: IDSA Guidelines for Management of Atypical Infections

1. Aspergillosis (IDSA Aspergillosis 2008)
   a. Epidemiology: Immunocompromised, neutropenia, advanced HIV, and inherited immunodeficiency and stem cell transplant
   b. Diagnosis
      i. Grows well on standard media for sputum culture; blood cultures of limited utility
      ii. May need invasive sampling
      iii. CT scan: Halo sign, air-crescent sign
      iv. Galactomannan EIA (specific) or 1,3-β-D-glucan (nonspecific)
   c. Treatment
      i. Start early treatment concurrent with evaluation
      ii. Voriconazole and amphotericin B doxycholate are the only licensed agents for treatment
      iii. Can also consider itraconazole, posaconazole, caspofungin in conjunction with infectious disease specialist
      iv. Decrease dose of steroids and other immunosuppressants if possible
      v. Hemoptysis requires emergent surgical evaluation
      vi. Surgical excision of lesion can be curative
      vii. Late management: Consider prophylaxis if planned for immunosuppression
      viii. Consider prophylaxis for the duration of immunosuppression
2. Blastomycosis (IDSA Blastomycosis 2008)
   a. Epidemiology: Occurs in midwest, southeast, south central US, and areas bordering Great Lakes and St. Lawrence seaway
   b. Treatment of pulmonary blastomycosis
      i. Severe: Amphotericin B (AmB) 3–5 mg/kg/day or AmB deoxycholate 0.7–1 mg/kg/day for 1–2 weeks, then itraconazole 200–400 mg TID × 3 days, then 200–400 mg BID × 6–12 months
      ii. Mild to moderate: Oral itraconazole 200–400 mg TID × 3 days, then daily to BID × 6–12 months
      iii. Follow serum itraconazole levels at 2 weeks to determine adequate levels
      iv. In setting of ARDS, consider steroids
3. Coccidioidomycosis (IDSA Coccidioidomycosis 2005)
   a. Epidemiology: "Valley fever" found in SW US; can reactivate in travelers; CAP that resolves after 1–3 weeks of infection; fatigue lasts weeks to months
   b. Presentation: Variable, from mild respiratory infection to progressive pulmonary destruction with metastatic emboli

c. Diagnosis
  i. Need to have a high suspicion, check anticoccidial antibodies from serum or sputum for all patients who are residents of or have traveled to an endemic region
  ii. Check for HIV in infected patients
d. Treatment
  i. Most mild-to-moderate cases resolve without treatment
  ii. Treat immunocompromised persons
  iii. Severe pneumonia
    1. Prolonged AmB deoxycholate 0.5–1.5 mg/kg/day or lipid AmB 2–5 mg/kg/day, ketoconazole 400 mg daily, fluconazole 400–800 mg/day or itraconazole 200 mg BID to TID
    2. More acute/rapid presentation, treat with AmB; subacute to chronic, treat with azole antifungal
    3. Other options: Voriconazole, posaconazole, caspofungin
  iv. Continue therapy at least 1 year versus indefinitely for immunocompromised persons
  v. Solitary nodule: Therapy or resection unnecessary; follow radiographically
4. *Cryptococcus* (IDSA 2010 *Cryptococcus*)
  a. Epidemiology: Opportunistic infection, generally immunocompromised host
  b. Diagnosis
    i. Antigen testing
    ii. Perform lumbar puncture (LP) in all immunocompromised hosts
    iii. Check for HIV for co-infection
  c. Treatment based on comorbid conditions
    i. Immunocompromised (HIV or organ transplant)
    ii. Mild-to-moderate infection: Fluconazole 400 mg/day oral × 6–12 months
    iii. For treatment of severe pneumonia, ARDS, or dissemination like CNS disease, consider steroids
    iv. HIV positive
      1. Induction with AmB deoxycholate 0.7–1 mg/kg/day
      2. If CD4 >100, *Cryptococcus* titer ≤1:512, stop fluconazole after 1 year
      3. Consider surgery for non-resolving lesions or persistent symptoms
  d. Immunocompetent, non-transplant host
    i. Consider LP if CNS symptoms or high titers
    ii. Mild to moderate: Fluconazole 400 mg/day oral × 6–12 months; persistent positive titers do not preclude cessation of therapy; alternatives include itraconazole, posaconazole, and voriconazole

    iii. Severe disease: Treat like CNS disease and consider steroids

    iv. Consider surgery for non-resolving lesions or persistent symptoms

Sources:

1. NICE 2016: National Guideline Centre. Pneumonia in adults: diagnosis and management. London (UK): National Institute for Health and Care Excellence (NICE); 2016. 26 p. (Clinical Guideline; no. 191). [https://www.nice.org.uk/guidance/cg191]

2. IDSA 2007: Mandell L, Wunderink R, Anzueto A, et al. Infectious Diseases Society of America/American Thoracic Society consensus guidelines on the management of community-acquired pneumonia in adults. Clin Infect Dis. 2007:S27–S72. [https://www.ncbi.nlm.nih.gov/pubmed/17278083]

3. IDSA 2008 Aspergillosis: Walsh T, Anaissie E, Denning D, et al. Treatment of aspergillosis: clinical practice guidelines of the Infectious Diseases Society of America. Clin Infect Dis. 2008:46:327–360. [http://www.idsociety.org/uploadedFiles/IDSA/Guidelines-Patient_Care/PDF_Library/Aspergillosis.pdf]

4. IDSA 2008 Blastomycosis: Chapman S, Dismukes W, Proia L, et al. Clinical practice guidelines for the management of blastomycosis: 2008 update by the Infectious Diseases Society of America. Clin Infect Dis. 2008:46:1801–1812. [http://www.idsociety.org/uploadedFiles/IDSA/Guidelines-Patient_Care/PDF_Library/Blastomycosis.pdf]

5. IDSA 2005: Galgiani J, Ampel N, Blair J, et al. Coccidioidomycosis. Clin Infect Dis. 2005; 41:1217–1223. [http://www.idsociety.org/uploadedFiles/IDSA/Guidelines-Patient_Care/PDF_Library/Coccidioidomycosis.pdf]

6. IDSA 2010: Perfect J, Dismukes W, Dromer F, et al. Clinical practice guidelines for the management of cryptococcal disease: 2010 update by the Infectious Diseases Society of America. Clin Infect Dis. 2010;50:291–322. [https://www.idsociety.org/uploadedfiles/idsa/guidelines-patient_care/pdf_library/cryptococcal.pdf]

7. Lim WS, van der Eerden MM, Laing R, et al. Defining community-acquired pneumonia severity on presentation to hospital: an international derivation and validation study. Thorax. 2003 May;58(5):377–382. [https://www.ncbi.nlm.nih.gov/pubmed/12728155]

8. For further reading on the utility of procalcitonin, please consider the following resources:

    a. Schuetz P, et al. Effect of procalcitonin based guidelines vs standard guidelines on antibiotic use in lower respiratory tract infections. JAMA. 2009;302:1059–1066. [https://www.ncbi.nlm.nih.gov/pubmed/19738090]

    b. Schuetz P, et al. Procalcitonin algorithms for antibiotic therapy decisions. Arch Intern Med. 2011;171(15). [https://www.ncbi.nlm.nih.gov/pubmed/21824946]

    c. De Jong E, et al. Efficacy and safety of procalcitonin guidance in reducing the duration of antibiotic treatment in critically ill patients:

a randomized, controlled, open-label trial. Lancet Infect Dis. 2016 Feb 29. Vol 16, No 7, p819–927. [https://www.ncbi.nlm.nih.gov/pubmed/26947523]

d. Schuetz P, et al. Role of procalcitonin in managing adult patients with respiratory tract infections. Chest. 2012;141(4):1063–1073. [http://journal.publications.chestnet.org/article.aspx?articleid=1206490]

e. Agarwal R, Schwartz DN. Procalcitonin to guide duration of antimicrobial therapy in intensive care units: a systematic review. Clin Infect Dis. 2011;53(4):379–387. [http://cid.oxfordjournals.org/content/53/4/379.full]

f. Prkno A, et al. Procalcitonin-guided therapy in intensive care unit patients with severe sepsis and septic shock. A systematic review and meta-analysis. Crit Care. 2013;17(6):R291. [https://www.ncbi.nlm.nih.gov/pubmed/24330744]

g. Zsolt B, et al. Can procalcitonin levels indicate the need for adjunctive therapies in sepsis? Int J Antimicrob Agents. 2015;46:S13–S18. [https://www.ncbi.nlm.nih.gov/pubmed/26607343]

9. Brechot N, et al. Procalcitonin to guide antibiotic therapy in the ICU. Int J Antimicrob Agents. 2015;46:S19–S24. [http://www.ijaaonline.com/issue/S0924-8579(15)X0015-X]

10. Hugle T, et al. Serum procalcitonin for discrimination between septic and non-septic arthritis. Clin Esp Rheumatol. 2008 May–Jun;26(3):453–456. [https://www.ncbi.nlm.nih.gov/pubmed/18578968]

COPD EXACERBATION

Initial Assessment

1. Investigations (NICE 2016)
   a. CBC, BMP, CXR, EKG, consider ABG
   b. Theophylline level if on theophylline
   c. Sputum culture if purulent sputum or risk factors for resistant pathogens
   d. Blood cultures if patient is febrile
   e. Procalcitonin, helpful in guiding the following (see Table 3-3):
      i. Stop antibiotic treatment with confirmed or highly suspected sepsis in the ICU
      ii. Start and stop antibiotic treatment with suspected bacterial infection in the emergency department
2. Diagnosis (GOLD 2017)
   a. Spirometry is required to make the diagnosis in the clinical context of dyspnea, chronic cough or sputum production and has a history of risk factors for the disease; post-bronchodilator $FEV1/FVC < 0.70$ confirms the presence of persistent airflow limitation

TABLE 3-4

MODIFIED MRC DYSPNEA SCALE TO ASSESS SEVERITY OF COPD	
Modified MRC Dyspnea scale	
Grade 0	Only breathless with strenuous exercise
Grade 1	Short of breath when hurrying on level ground
	Or short of breath walking up a slight hill
Grade 2	Walks slower on level ground than people of the same age because of breathlessness
	Or stops for breath when walking at own pace on level ground
Grade 3	Stops for breath after walking about 100 yards
	Or stops for breath after a few minutes on level ground
Grade 4	Too breathless to leave the house
	Or breathless when dressing or undressing

Source: From Stenton C. The MRC breathlessness scale. Occup Med (Lond). 2008 May;58(3):226–7; with permission.

      b. Controversy exists as to the benefit of universal screening

      c. Decreased FEV1 and FVC predict all-cause mortality independent of tobacco smoking

      d. Alpha-1 antitrypsin deficiency (AATD): Consider at least one test in all patients with a diagnosis of COPD; low concentration, less than 20%, is highly suggestive of homozygous deficiency; screen family members if positive

      e. GOLD grade of airflow limitation

         i. GOLD 1 (mild): FEV1 $\geq$ 80% predicted

        ii. GOLD 2 (moderate): 50% $\leq$ FEV1 < 80% predicted

       iii. GOLD 3 (severe): 30% FEV1 < 50% predicted

       iv. GOLD 4 (very severe): FEV1 < 30% predicted

      f. Assess severity of symptoms: Use either modified MRC dyspnea scale (Table 3-4) or CAT assessment (Figure 3-1)

      g. Use symptom score to assign ABCD status for combined assessment (Table 3-5)

   3. Workflow to establish COPD diagnosis

      a. Confirm diagnosis with spirometry: Post-bronchodilator FEV_1/FVC <0.7

      b. Assess airflow limitation: GOLD grade 1–4

      c. Assess symptoms and risk of exacerbation: Apply ABCD tool (Table 3-5)

      d. Example: FEV1/FVC <0.7; GOLD grade 2; group A

APPENDIX: CONTENT AND STRUCTURE OF THE FINAL CAT QUESTIONNAIRE

How is your COPD?

For each item below, place a mark (√) in the box that best describes your experience.

Example: I am very happy | 0 | √1 | 2 | 3 | 4 | 5 | I am very sad

			SCORE
I never cough	0 1 2 3 4 5	I cough all the time	☐
I have no phlegm (mucus) in my chest at all	0 1 2 3 4 5	My chest is completely full of phlegm (mucus)	☐
My chest does not feel tight at all	0 1 2 3 4 5	My chest feels Very tight	☐
When I walk up a hill or one flight of stairs I am not breathless	0 1 2 3 4 5	When I walk up a hill or one flight of stairs I am very breathless	☐
I am not limited doing any activities at home	0 1 2 3 4 5	I am very limited doing activities at home	☐
I am confident leaving my home despite my lung condition	0 1 2 3 4 5	I am not at all confident leaving my home because of my lung condition	☐
I sleep soundly	0 1 2 3 4 5	I don't sleep soundly because of my lung condition	☐
I have lots of energy	0 1 2 3 4 5	I have no energy at all	☐

SCORE ☐☐

FIGURE 3-1. CAT assessment for severity of COPD. (From Jones PW, et al. Eur Respir J. 2009;34(3):648–654; with permission.)

TABLE 3-5

ABDC ASSESSMENT TOOL

History of Exacerbations	Symptom Score	GOLD Group
No hospitalizations And <2 exacerbations	Low	A
	High	B
Hospitalization Or ≥2 exacerbations	Low	C
	High	D

"Low": mMRC 0–1 or CAT <10; "high": mMRC ≥2 or CAT ≥10.

Source: Adapted from GOLD 2017.

Acute Medical Management

1. Gauge severity (GOLD 2017)
   a. Mild: Treated with short-acting bronchodilators (SABDs) only
   b. Moderate: Treated with SABD + antibiotics and/or corticosteroids
   c. Severe: Patient requires hospitalization or visit to emergency room, may have acute respiratory failure
2. Determine respiratory status (GOLD 2017)
   a. No respiratory failure: RR: 20–30 breath/min, no accessory muscle use, no changes in mentation, hypoxemia improves with Venturi mask 28%–35% FiO_2; no increase in $PaCO_2$
   b. Acute respiratory failure, non-life-threatening: RR >30, use of accessory muscles, no change in mentation, hypoxemia improved with Venturi mask 25%–30% FiO_2, hypercarbia: $PaCO_2$ increased compared to baseline or 50–60 mmHg
   c. Acute respiratory failure, life-threatening: RR >30, use of accessory muscles, acute change in mentation, hypoxemia not improved with Venturi mask >40% FiO_2, hypercarbia: $PaCO_2$ increased compared to baseline or >60 mmHg or pH ≤7.25
3. Management
   a. Give SABD ± short-acting anticholinergic (GOLD 2017)
   b. Steroids
      i. Give to all hospitalized patients barring contraindication (NICE 2016)
      ii. Systemic corticosteroids (≤5–7 days) can improve lung function (FEV1), oxygenation and short recovery time, and hospitalization duration (GOLD 2017)
      iii. Dosing
      iv. Prednisone 40 mg PO daily ×5 days (GOLD 2017)
      v. Prednisolone 30 mg PO daily ×7–14 days (NICE 2016)
      vi. Oral therapy is as effective as intravenous (GOLD 2017)
   c. Antibiotics
      i. Can shorten recovery time, reduce risk of early relapse, treatment failure, and hospitalization duration (Evidence B) (GOLD 2017)
      ii. Antibiotics are only indicated in the case of purulent sputum or evidence of pneumonia (NICE 2016)
      iii. Give initial empiric treatment with penicillin, macrolide, or tetracycline (NICE 2016)
      iv. Use evidence from sputum culture and local antibiogram to guide therapy (NICE 2016)
   d. Oxygen: Administer to the individualized target range, usually 88–92% (refer to local protocols), leads to better outcomes versus high-flow oxygen; monitor pulse oximetry (NICE 2016)

e. Methylxanthines
   i. Do not use – Increased side effects profiles (GOLD 2017)
   ii. Only use intravenous theophylline with frequent monitoring as an adjunct to management of exacerbations of COPD when response to nebulized bronchodilators is inadequate (NICE 2016)
f. Delivery system (NICE 2016)
   i. Use nebulizers or handheld inhalers to administer therapy
   ii. Supervise patient in the use of the inhaler device; change to handheld inhalers as soon as condition has stabilized, as this may facilitate earlier hospital discharge
   iii. Use nebulizer if patient is hypercapnic or acidotic; use compressed air, not oxygen
g. Oxygen may be administered simultaneously via nasal cannula
4. Do not routinely monitor daily peak expiratory flow (PEF) or FEV1 (NICE 2016)

Interventions
1. ICU admission: Consider for the following reasons (GOLD 2017)
   a. Severe dyspnea with inadequate response to initial therapy
   b. Altered mentation
   c. Hypoxemia, PaO_2 <40 mmHg, or worsening acidosis, pH <7.25 despite supplemental oxygen and NIV
   d. Need for invasive mechanical ventilation
   e. Hemodynamic instability
2. Noninvasive ventilation[2]: Consider for the following reasons (GOLD 2017)
   a. Respiratory acidosis ($PaCO_2$ ≥45 and pH <7.35)
   b. Severe dyspnea with clinical signs suggesting respiratory muscle fatigue or increased work of breathing
   c. Persistent hypoxemia, despite supplemental O_2
3. Invasive mechanical ventilation: Consider for the following reasons (GOLD 2017)
   a. Unable to tolerate NIV or failure on NIV
   b. Status post respiratory or cardiac arrest
   c. Diminished consciousness or agitation
   d. Massive aspiration or persistent vomiting
   e. Severe hemodynamic instability, unresponsive to fluids
   f. Severe ventricular or supraventricular arrhythmia
   g. Life-threatening hypoxemia

---

[2]Use NIV as the first mode of ventilation use in COPD patients with acute respiratory failure who have no absolute contraindications because it improves gas exchange, reduces the work of breathing and the need for intubation, decreases hospitalization duration, and improves survival (GOLD 2017). It can also help with clearance of sputum (NICE 2016).

Management After Stabilization

1. Measure spirometry in all patients before discharge (NICE 2016)
2. Discharge criteria: Reestablish on optimal maintenance bronchodilator regimen and satisfactory oximetry or ABG (NICE 2016)
3. Follow-up within 1 month of discharge and attempt to modify exacerbating factors (GOLD 2017)
4. Smoking cessation (GOLD 2017)
   a. Greatest capacity due to influence natural history of COPD
   b. Use the Ask, Advise, Assess, Assist, and Arrange strategy
   c. Counseling for as little as 3 minutes improves cessation rates; there is a relationship between counseling intensity and cessation success
   d. Counseling plus either nicotine replacement therapy or antidepressants are effective (NICE 2016)
5. Vaccinations (GOLD 2017)
   a. PCV13 and PSSV23 for all patients ≥65 years old
   b. PSSV23 for COPD patients <65 years old to reduce the incidence of CAP
   c. PCV13 vaccination for patients ≥65 years old reduces bacteremia and serious invasive pneumococcal disease
   d. Influenza vaccine reduces serious illness and death in COPD patients
6. Pharmacology for stable COPD (GOLD 2017)
   a. See Table 3-6 for summary of interventions that reduce frequency of COPD exacerbations
   b. Give triple inhaled therapy of ICS + LAMA + LABA rather than ICS + LABA or LAMA monotherapy for patients with moderate-to-severe COPD[3]
   c. Give ICS + LABA in patients with moderate-to-severe COPD, rather than either component individually[4]
   d. Regular treatment with ICS increases risk of pneumonia
   e. Do not give long-term oral glucocorticoids[5]
   f. In patients with severe to very severe COPD and history of exacerbations
      i. PDE4 inhibitor improves lung function and reduces moderate and severe exacerbations
      ii. PDE4 inhibitor improves lung function and decreases exacerbations in patients who are on fixed dose LABA/ICS combinations
   g. Consider long-term azithromycin or erythromycin
      i. Reduces exacerbations over 1 year

---

[3] Improved lung function, symptoms, health status, and fewer exacerbations.
[4] Improved lung function, health status, and fewer exacerbations.
[5] Numerous side effects and no evidence of benefit.

TABLE 3-6

INTERVENTIONS THAT REDUCE FREQUENCY OF COPD EXACERBATIONS

Interventions that reduce frequency of COPD exacerbations

Bronchodilators	LABA
	LAMA
	LABA + LAMA
Corticosteroid regimens	LABA + ICS
	LABA + LAMA + ICS
Anti-inflammatory (nonsteroid)	Roflumilast
Anti-infectives	Vaccines
	Long-term macrolides
Mucoregulators	N-acetylcysteine
	Carbocysteine
Other	Smoking cessation
	Rehabilitation
	Lung volume reduction

Source: Adapted from GOLD 2017.

    ii. Azithromycin is associated with an increased incidence of bacterial resistance and hearing test impairments

  h. Consider NAC and carbocysteine; regular use reduces the risk of exacerbations in select populations

 i. Oxygen

    i. Give long-term oxygen to patients with severe chronic resting arterial hypoxemia for improved survival; criteria for long-term oxygen include:

      1. PaO_2 <55 mmHg

      2. SaO_2 <88%

      3. PaO_2 >55 but <60 mmHg with right heart failure or erythrocytosis

    ii. Titrate oxygen to SaO_2 ≥90%; reassess in 60–90 days

    iii. In patients with stable COPD and moderate resting or exercise-induced arterial desaturation, prescription of long-term oxygen does not lengthen time to death or first hospitalization or provide sustained benefit in health status or lung function in 6-minute walking distance

      iv. Adequate resting oxygenation at sea level does not exclude the development of severe hypoxemia when traveling by air

   j. NPPV may improve hospitalization free survival in selected patients after recent hospitalization, particularly in those with pronounced daytime persistent hypercapnia ($PaCO_2 \geq 52$ mmHg)

   k. Simvastatin does not prevent exacerbations in COPD patients at increased risk of exacerbations and without indications for statin therapy; observational studies suggest that statins may have positive effects on some outcomes in patients with COPD who receive them for cardiovascular and metabolic indications

   l. Leukotriene modifiers have not been tested adequately in COPD patients

   m. There is no conclusive evidence of beneficial role of antitussives in patients with COPD

   n. Vasodilators do not improve outcomes and may worsen oxygenation, other than as mentioned above with chronic pancreatitis

   o. Intravenous augmentation therapy for AATD may slow down the progression of emphysema

7. Other management (GOLD 2017)

   a. Pulmonary rehabilitation improves dyspnea, health status, and exercise tolerance in stable patients

   b. Pulmonary rehabilitation reduces hospitalizations among patients who have had a recent exacerbation within the prior 4 weeks (GOLD 2017, NICE 2016)

   c. Education alone on the pulmonary condition has not been shown to be effective

   d. Self-management intervention with communication with a health care professional improves health status and decreases hospitalizations and emergency department visits

   e. Integrated care and telehealth have not demonstrated benefit

   f. Consider palliative care evaluation for patients with a life expectancy of less than 6 months

Sources:

1. Global Strategy for the Diagnosis, Management and Prevention of COPD, Global Initiative for Chronic Obstructive Lung Disease (GOLD) 2017. [http://goldcopd.org/gold-2017-global-strategy-diagnosis-management-prevention-copd/]

2. Chronic Obstructive Pulmonary Disease: Evidence update 2012. National Institute for Health and Clinical Excellence (NICE). [https://www.nice.org.uk/guidance/cg101/evidence/evidence-update-pdf-134515693]

3. Managing Exacerbations of COPD Pathway. National Institute for Health and Clinical Excellence (NICE). 2016. [http://pathways.nice.org.uk/pathways/chronic-obstructive-pulmonary-disease/managing-exacerbations-of-copd]

4. Stenton, C. The MRC breathlessness scale. Occup Med. 2008;58(3):226–227. [https://www.academic.oup.com/occmed/article/58/3/226/1520518/]

5. Jones PW, Harding G, Berry P, et al. Development and first validation of the COPD assessment test. Eur Respir J. 2009;34(3):648–654. [https://www.ncbi.nlm.nih.gov/pubmed/19720809]

IDIOPATHIC PULMONARY FIBROSIS

Initial Assessment (NICE 2013)

1. Consider IPF in patients with persistent breathlessness on exertion, persistent cough, age over 45, bilateral inspiratory crackles, clubbing of the fingers, and normal or impaired spirometry usually with restrictive pattern but sometimes with an obstructive pattern

2. Evaluate for other possible etiologies of symptoms (e.g., congestive heart failure, pneumonia, coronary artery disease)

3. Perform chest radiograph, pulmonary function test, high-resolution lung CT for all patients with suspected IPF

4. Consider bronchoalveolar lavage, transbronchial biopsy, and/or surgical lung biopsy if diagnosis cannot be made confidently based on clinical features, lung function, and radiological findings

5. Consider performing 6-minute walk test, measuring distance and oxygen saturations, and quality of life assessment in all new diagnoses of IPF

6. Diagnosis and management requires pulmonologist, radiologist, interstitial lung disease nurse, pathologist, thoracic surgeon, and multidisciplinary team coordinator

Acute Medical Management

1. Oxygen therapy: Assess for need with pulse oximetry and 6-minute walk test (ATS 2011, NICE 2013)

2. Steroids: Give IV or oral steroids during exacerbation (prednisone 1 mg/kg/day or 1 g/day IV methylprednisolone, with taper) (ATS 2011)

3. Acid suppression: Give PPI or H2 blocker for all patients with IPF (ATS 2011, 2015, NICE 2013)

4. Disease-modifying pharmacotherapy: Initiate or continue nintedanib and pirfenidone (ATS 2015)

5. Mechanical ventilation: Do not routinely offer mechanical ventilation, including noninvasive, for life-threatening respiratory failure; IPF is a progressive disease, associated with poor outcomes even with mechanical ventilation (ATS 2011, 2015, NICE 2013)

6. Do not use the following therapies: Combination prednisone, azathioprine, and *N*-acetylcysteine; *N*-acetylcysteine monotherapy; ambrisentan; bosentan; macitentan; imatinib; sildenafil; and anticoagulation (ATS 2011, 2015, NICE 2013)

Interventions

1. Bronchoscopy, bronchoalveolar lavage, transbronchial biopsy, or surgical lung biopsy: Consider if diagnosis cannot be made confidently based on clinical features, lung function testing, and radiological findings (ATS 2011)

Management After Stabilization

1. Oxygen therapy: Assess for need based on dyspnea or oxygen saturation (NICE 2013)
2. Symptomatic management: Consider opioids, benzodiazepines for dyspnea at rest not relieved by oxygen; consider thalidomide for intractable cough (NICE 2013)
3. Acid suppression: H2 blocker or PPI indefinitely for all patients with IPF (NICE 2013, ATS 2015)
4. Disease-modifying pharmacotherapy: Continue nintedanib and pirfenidone when transitioned to outpatient therapy (NICE 2013, ATS 2015)
5. Pulmonary rehabilitation
   a. Consists of aerobic conditioning, strength and flexibility training, education, nutritional interventions, and psychosocial support (ATS 2011, 2015, NICE 2013)
   b. Reassess for need every 6–12 months (NICE 2013)
6. Tobacco cessation: Tobacco cessation in applicable patients (NICE 2013)
7. Lung transplantation: Refer for lung transplantation assessment if patients wish to explore lung transplantation and if there are no absolute contraindications (NICE 2013)
8. Palliative care: Consider referring patients with IPF for palliative care given progressive and fatal nature of disease (NICE 2013)

Sources:

1. ATS 2011: Raghu G, Collard HR, Egan JJ, et al. An official ATS/ERS/JRS/ALAT statement: idiopathic pulmonary fibrosis: evidence based guideline for diagnosis and management. Am J Respir Crit Care Med. 2011;183:788–824. [https://www.ncbi.nlm.nih.gov/pubmed/21471066]
2. ATS 2015: Raghu G, Rochwerg B, Zhang Y, et al. An official ATS/ERS/JRS/ALAT clinical practice guideline: treatment of idiopathic pulmonary fibrosis. Am J Respir Crit Care Med. 2015 June;192(2):3–19. [https://www.ncbi.nlm.nih.gov/pubmed/26177183]
3. NICE 2013: National Institute for Health and Care Excellence (NICE). Idiopathic pulmonary fibrosis in adults: diagnosis and management – clinical guideline. National Institute for Health and Care Excellence. June 12, 2013. [https://www.nice.org.uk/guidance/cg163]. Accessed February 01, 2017.

Neurology

Tipu V. Khan
Seth Alkire
Samantha Chirunomula

ACUTE ISCHEMIC STROKE

Initial Assessment (AHA/ASA 2013)

1. Establish "last normal" by determining time of symptom onset
2. Use a standardized stroke scale like the AHA/ASA 2018[1] to assess severity and help identify region of involvement
3. Get non-contrast CT head (if CT not available, get brain MRI) and blood glucose, within 20 minutes of presentation and prior to giving tPA. Get O_2 saturation, chemistry panel, CBC, markers for cardiac ischemia, PT/PTT, and an ECG, but do not delay tPA to obtain results.
4. Additional imaging
   a. Consider MRI with diffusion-weighted imaging in consultation with neurology, but do not obtain routinely.
   b. If symptoms persist, get intracranial vascular imaging such as CTA or MRA if candidate for rTPA or mechanical thrombectomy. Do not delay administration of rTPA to await vascular imaging. Do not delay CTA to await creatinine level.
   c. If symptoms have resolved, get intracranial vascular imaging such as CTA or MRA to exclude proximal vessel disease if results would alter management.
   d. In all patients suspected of TIA, get noninvasive imaging of cervical vessels.

Acute Medical Management (AHA/ASA 2013)

1. Antiplatelet agents
   a. Give oral aspirin 325 mg loading dose within the first 48 hours
   b. Do not routinely give early clopidogrel, tirofiban, and eptifibatide

---

[1] AHA/ASA 2018: Powers WJ, Rabinstein AA, Akerson T et. al. Guidelines for the early management of patients with acute ischemic stroke: A Guideline for Healthcare professionals from the American Heart Association/American Stroke Association. Stroke. 2018;49.

     c. Aspirin is not a substitute for other acute interventions, including rTPA

     d. Do not give aspirin as an adjunctive treatment to rTPA

2. Blood pressure

     a. If receiving rTPA

     b. Lower blood pressure to <185 mmHg systolic and <110 mmHg diastolic prior to giving rTPA

     c. Maintain <180/105 mmHg for at least 24 hours after rTPA

     d. If not receiving rTPA

     e. Do not lower blood pressure unless markedly elevated (i.e., >220/120)

     f. If markedly elevated, lower blood pressure by 15% during the first 24 hours

     g. Hold outpatient antihypertensive medications at admission for the first 24 hours

3. Anticoagulation: Do not routinely start anticoagulation urgently in the following clinical settings:

     a. Severe stenosis of an internal carotid artery ipsilateral to ischemic stroke

     b. Acute stroke, where the aim is to decrease neurologic worsening or improve outcomes

     c. Non-cerebrovascular conditions with indication for anticoagulation, as they increase the risk of serious intracranial hemorrhage

     d. Received rTPA in the previous 24 hours

4. Blood glucose[2]

     a. Correct hypoglycemia to blood glucose 60–180 mg/dL; frequent monitoring may be necessary, and intensive care may be appropriate

5. Volume/Cardiac status

     a. Correct hypovolemia with IV normal saline

     b. Correct cardiac arrhythmias that cause a decrease in output

6. Neuroprotective modalities

     a. Continue statins in patients who are already taking them at the time of stroke onset

     b. Hypothermia: Utility not well established

     c. Transcranial near-infrared laser therapy: Utility not well established

     d. Hyperbaric oxygen: Utility not well established, except for stroke secondary to air embolism

7. Positioning/Monitoring

---

[2]There is no data to support reducing hyperglycemia to improve stroke outcomes. There is real harm to hypoglycemia in stroke patients. Consider maintaining blood glucose 140–180 mg/dL, in accordance with American Diabetes Association guidelines for hospitalized patients.

a. Head of bed 15–30 degrees for patients at risk for obstruction, aspiration, or those with suspected elevated ICP
b. Supine if non-hypoxemic
c. Cardiac monitoring for at least 24 hours
d. Oxygen: Supplemental O_2 to maintain $O_2 > 94\%$

Interventions

1. rTPA (AHA/ASA 2013)
   a. See Table 4-1 for indications and contraindications
   b. <3 hours from symptom onset: Give rTPA 0.9 mg/kg IV for patients who have met selection criteria (see below for criteria); administer TPA as soon as possible, with the goal of door-to-needle time of 60 minutes
   c. 3–4.5 hours from symptom onset: Selection criteria are narrowed to exclude from rTPA therapy patients who are >80 years old, taking oral anticoagulants regardless of INR, baseline NIHSS score >25, imaging evidence of ischemic injury involving more than 1/3 of MCA territory or patients with history of stroke and diabetes
   d. Consider rTPA if patient has seizure and if evidence suggests that residual impairments are secondary to stroke and not postictal phenomenon

2. rTPA in specific populations (AHA/ASA 2016)
   a. Age >80: Do not withhold rTPA due to age alone; there is a significant treatment benefit despite a higher bleeding risk
   b. Severe stroke symptoms: Do not withhold rTPA for the risk of hemorrhagic transformation; the proven clinical benefit outweighs the risk
   c. Mild but disabling symptoms: Give rTPA; "disabling symptoms" is based on clinical judgment
   d. Mild symptoms: Explore risks and benefits with the patient before administering rTPA
   e. Patients with rapid improvement: rTPA is reasonable in patients with improving symptoms, but persistent moderate disability; do not withhold rTPA to await further improvement
   f. Pregnancy: Consider rTPA when anticipated benefits of treating moderate to severe symptoms outweigh anticipated risk of uterine bleeding
   g. Coagulopathy/Anticoagulant therapy
      i. Do not give rTPA if platelets <100k/microliter, INR>1.7, aPTT >40 seconds, PT >15 seconds
      ii. Consider rTPA in patients receiving VKA therapy with INR ≤1.7
      iii. Do not give rTPA if INR >1.7

CHAPTER 4

TABLE 4-1

ADMINISTRATION OF INTRAVENOUS RECOMBINANT TISSUE PLASMINOGEN ACTIVATOR (RTPA) FOR ACUTE ISCHEMIC STROKE (AIS)[1]

Indications	Contraindications
• Clinical diagnosis of stroke • Onset of symptoms to time of administration <4.5 hours[2] • CT scan showing no hemorrhage or edema of >1/3 of the MCA territory • Age 18+ years • Consent by patient or surrogate	• Sustained BP >185/110 mmHg despite treatment • Platelets <100,000; HCT <25%; glucose <50 or >400 mg/dL • Use of heparin within 48 hours and prolonged PTT, or elevated INR • Rapidly improving symptoms • Prior stroke or head injury within 3 months; prior intracranial hemorrhage • Major surgery in preceding 14 days • Minor stroke symptoms • Gastrointestinal bleeding in preceding 21 days • Recent myocardial infarction • Coma or stupor

Administration of rtPA

IV access with two peripheral IV lines (avoid arterial or central line placement)
Review eligibility for rtPA
Administer 0.9 mg/kg IV (maximum 90 mg) IV as 10% of total dose by bolus, followed by remainder of total dose over 1 hour
Frequent cuff blood pressure monitoring
No other antithrombotic treatment for 24 hours
For decline in neurologic status or uncontrolled blood pressure, stop infusion, give cryoprecipitate, and reimage brain emergently
Avoid urethral catheterization for ≥2 hours

[1]See Activase (tissue plasminogen activator) package insert for complete list of contraindications and dosing.
[2]Depending on the country, IV rtPA may be approved for up to 4.5 hours with additional restrictions.
BP, blood pressure; CT, computed tomography; HCT, hematocrit; INR, international normalized ratio; MCA, middle cerebral artery; PTT, partial thromboplastin time.
Source: Smith WS, et al: Cerebrovascular diseases. In: Kasper DL, et al. (eds). *Harrison's Principles of Internal Medicine,* 19th ed. New York: McGraw-Hill, 2015, Table 446–1.

    iv. Do not give rTPA if LMWH in the preceding 24 hours
    v. Do not give rTPA to patients who have taken direct factor Xa inhibitors or direct thrombin inhibitors in the last 48 hours (assuming normal renal function), unless normal lab tests such as aPTT, INR, platelet count, direct factor Xa activity, ecarin clotting time are obtained

h. Major surgery/Major trauma
   i. Consider rTPA carefully if surgery or major trauma in the preceding 14 days
   ii. Do not give rTPA if severe head injury within 3 months
   iii. Do not give rTPA if intracranial/spinal surgery within 3 months
i. Acute MI
   i. Consider rTPA for cerebral ischemia followed by PCA for myocardial ischemia in patients with concurrent ischemic stroke and MI
   ii. Give rTPA to patients with any NSTEMI or STEMI involving inferior or right infarction
   iii. Consider rTPA if STEMI involving anterior wall
j. Other cardiac conditions
   i. Pericarditis or left thrombus: Give rTPA if major disability from stroke
   ii. Endocarditis: Do not give rTPA
k. Recent ischemic stroke: Avoid rTPA if stroke in past 3 months
l. Active internal bleeding
   i. Do not give rTPA if structural GI malignancy or bleed in the past 21 days
   ii. Consider rTPA in setting of more remote GI/GU bleeds
m. Arterial puncture: Uncertain safety of rTPA if arterial puncture in noncompressible area within 7 days
n. Aneurysm: May consider rTPA if known unruptured and unsecured intracranial aneurysm <10 mm
o. AVM: Known unruptured and untreated intracranial vascular malformation – Risks and usefulness of rTPA not established; may be considered in patients with severely disabling symptoms
p. Intracranial neoplasms
   i. Known extra-axial: rTPA is probably helpful
   ii. Known intra-axial: rTPA is potentially harmful
q. Medical comorbidities
   i. ESRD: May give rTPA if aPTT normal; if aPTT abnormal, risk of hemorrhage is elevated
   ii. Systemic malignancy: May give rTPA if life expectancy is >6 months

Management After Stabilization (AHA/ASA 2013)

1. Institutional measures
   a. Use specialized stroke care units with incorporated rehabilitation
   b. Transfer patients with major infarctions at risk of malignant brain edema to a center with neurosurgery expertise
2. Prevention of complications
   a. Give subcutaneous anticoagulants to prevent venous thromboembolism
   b. If anticoagulation is contraindicated, use aspirin to prevent venous thromboembolism

c. Do not give therapeutic anticoagulation routinely

d. Assess swallowing before advancing diet

e. Give enteral feeds if unable to take solid foods or liquids orally; use nasoduodenal, PEG, or NG tubes while undergoing efforts to restore the ability to swallow; preferentially use NG tubes for the first 2–3 weeks before undergoing PEG tube placement

f. Mobilize patients early if able

g. Do not give corticosteroids for brain edema caused by ischemic stroke

Sources:

1. AHA/ASA 2013: Jauch EC, Saver JL, Adams HP, et al. Guidelines for the early management of patients with acute ischemic stroke: a guideline for healthcare professionals from the American Heart Association/American Stroke Association. Stroke. 2013;44(3):870–947. [http://stroke.ahajournals.org/content/44/3/870]

2. AHA/ASA 2016: Demaerschalk BM, Kleindorfer DO, Adeoye OM, et al. Scientific rationale for the inclusion and exclusion criteria for intravenous alteplase in acute ischemic stroke: a statement for healthcare professionals from the American Heart Association/American Stroke Association. Stroke. 2016;47:581–641. [http://stroke.ahajournals.org/content/47/2/581]

ACUTE HEMORRHAGIC STROKE

Acute Medical Management

1. General measures (AHA/ASA 2015)

   a. Monitor all patients with ICH in the ICU

   b. Avoid hypoglycemia; maintain normoglycemia

   c. Use normal saline for maintenance fluids and avoid hypotonic fluids to prevent cerebral edema

2. Anticoagulation (AHA/ASA 2015)

   a. Stop all anticoagulation at time of diagnosis of ICH

   b. If patient is on warfarin, correct coagulopathies with vitamin K, PCC, and other factors as needed; PCC may be superior to FFP as there are fewer associated complications and the correction of INR is more rapid

   c. If patient is on heparin, consider protamine sulfate

   d. Consider FEIBA, PCCs, rFVIIa on individual basis for reversal of coagulopathy in patients taking rivaroxaban, dabigatran, and apixaban

   e. In patients with DVT or PE, consider systemic anticoagulation or IVC filter

3. Blood products (AABB 2015)

   a. Platelet transfusion has not been demonstrated to benefit patients on antiplatelet medications

b. Give platelet transfusion if thrombocytopenia is present

c. Insufficient evidence to support or refuse the general use of platelets in patients with ICH

4. Thromboprophylaxis (AHA/ASA 2015)

 a. Give sequential compression devices unless contraindicated

 b. Consider LMWH or unfractionated heparin in immobilized patients 1–4 days after stroke onset once cessation of bleeding has been documented

5. Blood pressure (AHA/ASA 2015)

 a. If SBP is between 150 and 220 mmHg, lower SBP to 140 mmHg acutely if no contraindication

 b. If SBP is over 220 mmHg, consider aggressive reduction of BP with continuous IV infusion and frequent BP monitoring

6. Seizure (AHA/ASA 2015)

 a. Do not give anti-epileptics routinely

 b. Perform continuous EEG in patients with depressed mental status out of proportion to the degree of brain injury

 c. Treat clinically evident seizures

7. Intracranial pressure management (AHA/ASA 2015)

 a. Elevate head of bed to 30 degrees once patient is euvolemic

 b. Give adequate analgesia and sedation, especially in intubated patients; avoid excessive sedation, which would prevent neurologic assessment and monitoring

 c. Consider paralysis with neuromuscular blockade to reduce ICP in patients not responding to sedation and analgesia alone

 d. Do not use glucocorticoids to lower ICP

 e. In patients with GCS <8, consider invasive monitoring and surgical treatment of ICP if there is evidence of transtentorial herniation, significant hydrocephalus, or intraventricular hemorrhage; CPP goal is 50–70 mmHg

 f. Medications to lower ICP

  i. Give IV mannitol to lower ICP quickly and effectively; titrate to plasma hyperosmolality of 300–310 mOsm/kg while maintaining adequate plasma volume; avoid hypovolemia and hyperosmotic state

  ii. If mannitol fails, consider barbiturate sedation; titrate to EEG measured burst-suppression pattern of electrical activity

 g. $PaCO_2$ goal: 25–30 mmHg

8. Preventing long-term complications

Management After Stabilization (AHA/ASA 2015)

1. Blood pressure goal: <130/80 mmHg long term

2. Antiplatelets and anticoagulation

a. Consider resuming antiplatelet therapy after any ICH; optimal timing not established, but likely safe in the days following ICH
b. Avoid oral anticoagulation for at least 4 weeks in patients without mechanical heart valves; optimal timing to resume oral anticoagulation after an anticoagulant-related ICH is uncertain
c. If warfarin-associated nonlobar ICH and strong indication for anticoagulation, consider resuming warfarin after 4 weeks
d. If warfarin-associated spontaneous lobar ICH in patient with nonvalvular atrial fibrillation, do not give long-term anticoagulation
3. Rehabilitation: All patients with ICH should have access to multidisciplinary rehabilitation; start as early as possible and continue in the community as part of a well-coordinated program of accelerated hospital discharge and home-based resettlement

Sources:

1. AHA/ASA 2015: Hemphill JC, Greenberg SM, Anderson CS, et al. Guidelines for the management of spontaneous intracerebral hemorrhage: a guideline for healthcare professionals from the American Heart Association/American Stroke Association. Stroke. 2015;46(7):2032–2060. [https://www.ncbi.nlm.nih.gov/pubmed/26022637]
2. AABB 2015: Platelet transfusion: a clinical practice guideline from the AABB. JAMA. 2015;162(3):206–213. [https://www.ncbi.nlm.nih.gov/pubmed/25383671]

BACTERIAL MENINGITIS

Initial Assessment (IDSA 2004)

1. Suspect bacterial meningitis in patients with fever, headache, nuchal rigidity, and/or altered mental status

Acute Medical Management (IDSA 2004)

1. Follow management algorithm below
2. Send CSF for the following diagnostic tests:
   a. Gram stain and bacterial culture
   b. Cell count and differential
   c. Glucose
   d. Protein
   e. Opening pressure
3. Initiate empiric antibiotic therapy with the following:
   a. Ceftriaxone IV 2 g q12 hours
   b. Vancomycin IV 30–45 mg/kg/day divided q8–12 hours
      i. A loading dose of vancomycin IV 25–30 mg/kg may be used to rapidly achieve target concentration in seriously ill patients
      ii. Target vancomycin trough is 15–20 µg/mL

    c. For adults >50 years old or immunocompromised, add ampicillin IV 2 g q4 hours[3]

    d. If allergic to beta-lactams

       i. Replace ceftriaxone with moxifloxacin IV 400 mg q24 hours

       ii. Replace ampicillin with trimethoprim-sulfamethoxazole 5 mg/kg (trimethoprim component) IV q6–12 hours

4. Give corticosteroids: 0.15 mg/kg dexamethasone q6 hours for 2–4 days; ideally, give 10–20 minutes before or at least concomitant with initiation of antibiotic therapy

Management After Stabilization (IDSA 2004)

1. Diagnose bacterial meningitis based on CSF profile

    a. Opening pressure: 200–500 mm H_2O

    b. WBC: 1000–5000 with 80%–95% neutrophils

    c. CSF glucose: <40 mg/dL

2. Tailor antibiotic therapy based on CSF Gram stain if possible

3. Follow blood and CSF cultures and tailor antibiotic/antiviral therapy to target isolated pathogens

Source:

1. IDSA 2004: Tunkel A R, Hartman BJ, Kaplan SL, et al. Practice guidelines for the management of bacterial meningitis. Clin Infect Dis. 2004;39(9):1267–1284. [https://academic.oup.com/cid/article-lookup/39/9/1267]

ENCEPHALITIS

Initial Assessment (IDSA 2008)

1. Suspect acute encephalitis in patients with fever, headache, altered level of consciousness, behavioral changes, focal neurologic signs, and seizures

2. Perform laboratory workup including:

    a. CBC

    b. Creatinine

    c. Transaminases

    d. PT/INR, PTT

    e. Chest X ray

    f. Neuroimaging (MRI preferred over CT, but do not delay imaging to obtain MRI)

3. Lumbar puncture with CSF culture (see Table 4-2 for interpretation parameters)

---

[3] Primarily to provide coverage for *Listeria* infection.

Acute Medical Management (IDSA 2008)

1. Start empiric acyclovir immediately if viral encephalitis suspected
   a. 10 mg/kg IV q8 hours in children and adults with normal renal function
   b. 20 mg/kg IV q8 hours in neonates
2. Give appropriate therapy for presumed bacterial meningitis if clinically indicated (see Figure 4-1 for initial management)
3. If there are clinical clues suggestive of rickettsial or ehrlichial infection during the appropriate season, add doxycycline to empiric regimen

Management After Stabilization (IDSA 2008)

1. Once pathogen has been identified, select a treatment specifically for that pathogen
2. Consider acute disseminated encephalomyelitis in all patients; if suspicion is high, treat with high-dose IV corticosteroids (i.e., methylprednisolone, 1 g IV daily for at least 3–5 days)

TABLE 4-2

TYPICAL CSF PARAMETERS FOR VARIOUS INFECTIONS			
	Bacterial	**Viral**	**Fungal/TB**
Color	Turbid	Clear	Clear
Opening pressure	High	Normal or mildly increased	High
Glucose	Low	Low	Normal
Serum: CSF glucose ratio	<0.4	>0.6	<0.4
Protein	High	Normal	Normal to elevated
WBC count	>500	<1000	100–500
WBC differential	Predominantly PMNs	Increased lymphocytes	Increased lymphocytes

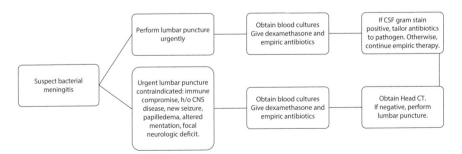

FIGURE 4-1. Initial management of bacterial meningitis. (From IDSA 2004; with permission.)

3. Perform plasma exchange in individuals who respond poorly to corticosteroids

Source:

1. IDSA 2008: Tunkel AR, Glaser CA, Bloch KC, et al. The management of encephalitis: clinical practice guidelines by the Infectious Diseases Society of America. Clin Infect Dis. 2008;47(3):303–327. [https://academic.oup.com/cid/article/47/3/303/313455]

TRANSVERSE MYELITIS

Initial Assessment

1. Determine underlying etiology (AAN 2011)
   a. Idiopathic
      i. Usually there is a preceding GI, respiratory, or systemic illness (Curr Neurol Neurosci Rep. 2006)
   b. Secondary
      i. MS, para-infectious myelitis, lupus, Guillain-Barré syndrome, other systemic diseases
      ii. Often the initiating complaint of a new MS diagnosis
      iii. If it involves three or more vertebral segments, often due to neuromyelitis optica
2. Workup: Exclude compressive cord lesion
   a. Lumbar puncture
      i. Elevated CSF WBC of >10 cells/mm^3
      ii. Get oligoclonal bands, DRL, IgG index, cytology, and routine spinal studies
   b. MRI with and without gadolinium of the entire spine and brain
   c. Serum: NMO-IgG
   d. Diagnosis requires either pleocytosis of CSF or elevated IgG index or gadolinium enhancement on MRI
   e. Other workup
      i. TSH, auto-immune labs such as ANA/RF, ESR, CRP, rule out vascular myelopathies, metabolic and nutritional myelopathies, neoplasm, and radiation myelitis
3. Type
   a. Acute complete (ACTM)
   b. Acute partial (APTM)
      i. Higher risk of transition to MS; may be up to 90% in those with abnormal brain MRI

Acute Medical Management (AAN 2011)

1. Give high-dose burst steroids for 3–5 days

a. Methylprednisolone 1000 mg daily

b. Dexamethasone 200 mg daily

2. Longer steroid treatment may be needed, tailored to the patient's disease activity and guided by expert consultation

3. If motor impairment is present, consider plasma exchange: Five treatments of 1.1–1.5 plasma volumes every other day for 10 days

4. If severe TM, consider cyclophosphamide 800–1200 mg/m^2 once

Chronic Medical Management

1. Consider chronic immunomodulatory therapy for patients with recurrent disease

a. Azathioprine: 150–200 mg/daily

b. Methotrexate: 15–20 mg/week

c. Mycophenolate: 2–3 g/day

Management After Stabilization

1. Relapse higher with APTM

2. Idiopathic TM usually has at least a partial recovery but may take 1–6 months (J Child Neurol. 2003); ensure good PT/OT

3. Rapid onset or infectious causes tend to yield a prolonged (over years) recovery or permanent disability

Sources:

1. Scott TF, Frohman EM, De Seze J, et al. Evidence-based guideline: clinical evaluation and treatment of transverse myelitis. Neurology. 2011;77(24): 2128–2134. [http://www.neurology.org/content/77/24/2128.full.html]

2. Krishnan C, Kaplin AI, Pardo CA, et al. Demyelinating disorders: update on transverse myelitis. Curr Neurol Neurosci Rep. 2006;6(3):236–243. [https://www.ncbi.nlm.nih.gov/pubmed?term=16635433]

3. Defrense P, Hollenberg H, Husson B, et al. Acute transverse myelitis in children: clinical course and prognostic factors. J Child Neurol. 2003;18(6):401–406. [https://www.ncbi.nlm.nih.gov/pubmed/12886975]

ICU DELIRIUM

Identification (SCCM 2013)

1. Risk factors for delirium (SCCM 2013)

a. Preexisting dementia

b. History of hypertension

c. History of alcoholism

d. High severity of illness at admission

e. Comatose

2. Monitor all ICU patients routinely for delirium using a validated tool such as CAM-ICU or ICDSC

Prevention

1. Early mobilization
2. Daily sedation interruption or use lightest level of sedation possible using an analgesia-first sedation technique
3. Orientation protocols
4. Cognitive stimulation with visitors
5. Optimize sleep environment
6. Avoid problematic medications
   a. Benzodiazepines, opiates, propofol, epidural analgesia, analgosedatives are known triggers and should be avoided (CCM 2015)

Outcome

1. May take weeks to months to resolve
2. May worsen dementia disease state
3. Associated with increased short- and long-term mortality

Sources:

1. SCCM 2013: Barr J, Fraser GL, Puntillo K, et al. American College of Critical Care Medicine. Clinical practice guidelines for the management of pain, agitation, and delirium in adult patients in the intensive care unit. Crit Care Med. 2013;41(1):263–306. [https://www.guideline.gov/summaries/summary/43903?]
2. Zaal IJ, Devlin JW, Peelen LM, Slooter AJ. A systematic review of risk factors for delirium in the ICU. Crit Care Med. 2015;43(1):40–47. [https://www.ncbi.nlm.nih.gov/pubmed/25251759]

ICU AGITATION

Prevention (SCCM 2013)

1. Aim for light levels of sedation; lighter levels of sedation yield better patient outcomes and shorter ICU stays; use a validated sedation tool such as RASS or SAS (goal RASS –2 to 0)
2. Sedative choice: Non-benzodiazepine preferred over benzodiazepine (i.e., propofol or dexmedetomidine)

Acute Management (SCCM 2013)

1. Non-pharmacologic
   a. Reorientation
   b. Physical restraints
2. Pharmacologic
   a. Give atypical antipsychotics such as haloperidol, quetiapine, risperidone, ziprasidone, or olanzapine
      i. Watch QTc
      ii. Watch for extrapyramidal symptoms

Gastroenterology

Jacob A. David
John Paul Kelada

5

Initial Assessment

1. Consider discharge from ER and outpatient EGD if all criteria are met
   a. ACG 2012: BUN <18.2 mg/dL, Hg >13 g/dL (men) or 12 g/dL (women), systolic BP ≥110 mmHg, pulse <100 bpm, and no history of melena, syncope, cardiac failure, liver disease
   b. NICE 2012: If Blatchford score is 0 (BUN <18.6 mg/dL, Hgb ≥13 g/dL for males or ≥12 g/dL for females, systolic blood pressure ≥110 mmHg, HR <100, no melena, syncope, hepatic disease, heart failure)
2. Perform Endoscopy
   a. AASLD 2007, WGO 2013: Within 12 hours
   b. NICE 2012: Within 24 hours or immediately after resuscitation if unstable
   c. ACG 2012: Within 24 hours or 12 hours if unstable

Acute Medical Management

1. Antibiotic prophylaxis for variceal bleeding (AASLD 2007, WGO 2013)
   a. Give fluoroquinolone or cephalosporin for 7 days[1]
2. Somatostatin/somatostatin analogues (AASLD 2007, NICE 2012, WGO 2013)
   a. Start at presentation
      i. AASLD: Somatostatin, octreotide, vapreotide, or terlipressin
      ii. NICE: Terlipressin (not available in the United States)
      iii. WGO: Terlipressin or somatostatin preferred over somatostatin analogues
3. PPI for non-variceal bleeding

---

[1] AASLD and WGO: Norfloxacin 400 mg PO BID, IV ciprofloxacin, or ceftriaxone 1 g/24 h if advanced cirrhosis or high prevalence of quinolone-resistant organisms. NICE recommends antibiotic therapy but does not recommend specific antibiotics.

a. ACG: Start PPI at presentation: 80 mg IV bolus + 8 mg/h infusion ×72 hours[2] (ACG 2012)
b. NICE: Don't give PPI before endoscopy; give PPI after endoscopy if evidence of recent non-variceal bleeding (NICE 2012)

4. Resuscitative measures
   a. Hemoglobin transfusion threshold
      i. AASLD: <8 g/dL (AASLD 2007)
      ii. ACG: ≤7 g/dL; higher if evidence of intravascular volume depletion or comorbidities (i.e., coronary artery disease) (ACG 2012)
      iii. NICE, WGO: No specific goal (NICE 2012, WGO 2013)
   b. Other blood products
      i. If actively bleeding (NICE 2012)
         1. Transfuse platelets if <50k
         2. Transfuse fresh frozen plasma if INR >1.5× normal with subsequent cryoprecipitate if not at goal
         3. Give prothrombin complex if on warfarin
   c. Other resuscitative measures (WGO 2013)
      i. Consider tracheal intubation if acute or massive variceal bleeding to avoid bronchial aspiration of food or blood

Interventions

1. Balloon tamponade (AASLD 2007, WGO 2013)
   a. As temporizing measure ×24 hours while awaiting TIPS or endoscopic therapy
2. Therapeutic EGD for endoscopic variceal ligation or sclerotherapy (AASLD 2007, ACG 2012, NICE 2012, WGO 2013)
   a. First-line therapy
   b. ACG 2012: Repeat EGD up to two times for persistent bleeding
3. TIPS (AASLD 2007, NICE 2012, WGO 2013)
   a. If bleeding not controlled with EGD
   b. Child A or Child B with recurrent variceal hemorrhage
   c. NICE: If esophageal variceal bleeding not controlled by band ligation
   d. WGO: If bleeding is uncontrolled or recurring despite EGD and pharmacotherapy
4. Other procedures
   a. ACG 2012: Transcatheter arterial embolization or surgery if refractory bleeding
   b. NICE 2012: Interventional radiology preferably over surgery if rebleed after EGD

---

[2]PPI pre-endoscopy reduces the number of patients who have high-risk stigmata and require endoscopic therapy, but has not been shown to improve clinical outcomes.

Management After Stabilization

1. Non-selective beta blockers
   a. Start propranolol or nadolol 24 hours after stabilization (AASLD 2007)
   b. Adjust to maximal dose (25% of resting heart rate reduction up to 55 bpm) (WGO 2013)
2. Isosorbide 5-mononitrate
   a. AASLD 2007: Consider giving with beta blocker (small benefit; often poorly tolerated due to hypotension and renal hypoperfusion)
   b. WGO 2013: Don't use routinely; consider for young patients, Child-Pugh A, if failed sclero- and pharmacotherapy
3. Liver transplant referral
   a. AASLD 2007: Refer if Child-Pugh ≥ 7 or MELD ≥ 15
   b. WGO 2013: Refer if recurrent bleed or Child-Pugh B or C
4. Adjusting other medications
   a. Aspirin (ACG 2012)
      i. For secondary prevention, restart within 7 days, ideally 1–3
      ii. For primary prevention, discontinue or take in conjunction with PPI
      iii. NICE 2012: For secondary prevention, restart when hemostasis achieved
   b. NSAIDs
      i. ACG 2012: Discontinue or take in conjunction with PPI
      ii. NICE 2012: Discontinue during acute phase
   c. Other medications (NICE 2012)
      i. Consider discontinuing antiplatelet agents
      ii. Consider whether acid-suppressing drugs for primary prevention are necessary upon discharge from critical care or hospital
5. Proton pump inhibitors after endoscopy in non-variceal bleeding (ACG 2012)
   a. If high risk (active bleeding, visible vessel, or adherent clot) give continuous PPI infusion for 72 hours
   b. If low risk (clean-based or flat pigmented ulcer) can discharge same day with once-daily PPI
6. Somatostatin/somatostatin analogues after endoscopy in variceal bleeding
   a. AASLD 2007: Continue 3–5 days
   b. NICE 2012: Continue until definitive hemostasis or for 5 days
   c. WGO 2013: Continue 2–5 days

Sources:

1. AASLD 2007: Garcia-Tsao G, Sanyal, AJ, Grace ND, et al. Prevention and management of gastroesophageal varices and variceal hemorrhage in cirrhosis. Hepatology. 2007;46(3):922–938. [https://www.ncbi.nlm.nih.gov/pubmed/17879356]

2. ACG 2012: Laine L, Jensen DM. ACG practice guidelines: management of patients with ulcer bleeding. Am J Gastroenterol. 2012;107:345–360. [http://gi.org/guideline/management-of-patients-with-ulcer-bleeding/]
3. NICE 2012: National Institute for Health and Care Excellent. Acute upper gastrointestinal bleeding over 16s: management. 2012 June 13. [https://www.nice.org.uk/Guidance/CG141]
4. WGO 2013. Labrecque D, Khan AG, et al. WGO global guidelines: esophageal varices. 2014 January. [http://www.worldgastroenterology.org/guidelines/global-guidelines/esophageal-varices/esophageal-varices-english]

ASCITES

Initial Assessment (AASLD 2012)

1. Perform diagnostic paracentesis for
   a. new-onset ascites
   b. every hospitalization with history of ascites
2. Ascitic fluid analysis
   a. Send fluid for: Cell count + differential, total protein, and SAAG
      i. If suspicion for secondary peritonitis and PMNs are >250, distinguish secondary peritonitis from SBP by sending for the following: Protein, LDH, glucose, Gram stain, CEA, alkaline phosphatase[3]
   b. Culture the fluid at bedside (aerobic + anaerobic) when
      i. infection suspected
      ii. prior to initiation of antibiotics
3. Routine use of fresh frozen plasma for paracentesis is unnecessary

Acute Medical Management (AASLD 2012)

1. Albumin
   a. Give 1.5 g/kg within 6 hours and 1 g/kg on post-procedure day #3 if creatinine >1 mg/dL, BUN >30 mg/dL, or total bilirubin >4 mg/dL
   b. After large-volume paracentesis (>4 or 5 L), give 6–8 g per liter of fluid
2. Antibiotics
   a. Cefoxitin (2 g q8 hours, or other third-generation cephalosporin)
      i. Give if suspecting SBP (ascitic fluid PMNs >250 cells/mm^3 and fever or abdominal pain) while awaiting culture results

---

[3]Secondary peritonitis suggested when (1) CEA >5 ng/mL, ascitic fluid alkaline phosphatase >240 units/L or (2) multiple organisms on Gram stain and culture and two or more of the following: total protein >1 g/dL, lactate dehydrogenase greater than upper limit of normal for serum, glucose <50 mg/dL.

     ii. Change antibiotic based on local susceptibilities if patient recently received beta-lactam antibiotics

     iii. Can use oral ofloxacin if no prior exposure to quinolones, vomiting, shock, serum creatinine >3, or hepatic encephalopathy grade II+

Interventions (AASLD 2012)

1. Therapeutic paracentesis
   a. Perform for tense ascites
   b. Subsequently initiate sodium restriction and oral diuretics
2. Refer to surgery for secondary peritonitis
3. Repeat paracentesis
   a. For signs, symptoms, or laboratory evidence of developing infection
   b. To help distinguish between SBP and secondary peritonitis (after 48 hours)
   c. To assess treatment and response of PMN count and culture (after 48 hours) if initial PMNs >250 and/or recent beta-lactam antibiotic exposure and/or result of atypical culture and/or atypical response to antibiotics

Management After Stabilization (AASLD 2012)

1. Prophylactic antibiotics
   a. Give norfloxacin or trimethoprim/sulfamethoxazole daily for all patients after SBP
   b. Consider prophylaxis in patients high risk for SBP (ascitic fluid protein <1.5 g/dL and Cr ≥1.2, serum Na ≤130, or liver failure (Child score ≥9 and bilirubin ≥3)
   c. Give antibiotics (IV ceftriaxone or BID PO norfloxacin) in all patients with cirrhosis and GI bleed
2. Encourage cessation of alcohol
   a. Prescribe baclofen to reduce cravings
3. Fluid management
   a. Sodium restrict to 2 g per day
   b. Spironolactone, with or without the use of furosemide
   c. The above are preferred over serial therapeutic paracentesis
4. Avoid NSAIDs
5. Refractory ascites
   a. Midodrine improves survival
   b. Avoid ACEi/ARBs given risk of hypotension
   c. Refer for transplant
   d. Consider TIPS
   e. Consider peritoneovenous shunt for those who are not candidates for paracenteses, TIPS, or transplant
6. Refer for evaluation for transplant

Source:
1. AASLD 2012: Runyon B. AASLD practice guideline: introduction to the revised American Association for the study of liver disease practice guideline management of adult patients with ascites due to cirrhosis 2012. Hepatology. 2013 April;57(4). [https://www.aasld.org/sites/default/files/guideline_documents/AASLDPracticeGuidelineAsciteDuetoCirrhosis Update2012Edition4_.pdf]

HEPATIC ENCEPHALOPATHY

Initial Assessment (AASLD 2014)
1. Diagnose after excluding other causes of brain dysfunction
2. Increased ammonia does not aid in diagnosis, staging, or prognostic indication; normal value suggests reevaluation

Acute Medical Management (AASLD 2014)
1. Lactulose
   a. 25 mL q1–2 hours until 2+ soft bowel movements per day
   b. Goal: 2–3 soft bowel movements per day
2. Consider oral branched-chain amino acids or IV L-ornithine L-aspartate as alternative or additional therapy if patients nonresponsive to lactulose
3. Alternative choices include neomycin, metronidazole

Management After Stabilization (AASLD 2014)
1. Secondary prophylaxis
   a. Use lactulose routinely
   b. Give rifaximin as adjunct to lactulose if refractory
   c. Do not give prophylaxis routinely after post-transjugular intrahepatic portosystemic shunt (TIPS)
   d. Consider discontinuing prophylaxis if precipitating factors have been well controlled (i.e., infections, variceal bleeding), or liver function or nutritional status has improved
   e. Offer small meals or liquid nutritional supplements throughout the day as well as a late-night snack; consider oral branched-chain amino acids if patients unable to meet dietary protein needs
   f. Refer for transplant if recurrent intractable disease in the setting of liver failure

Source:
1. AASLD 2014: Vilstrup H, Amodio P, et al. AASLD: Hepatic encephalopathy in chronic liver disease: 2014 practice guideline by AASLD and EASL. 2014. [https://www.aasld.org/sites/default/files/guideline_documents/hepaticencephenhanced.pdf]

ALCOHOLIC HEPATITIS

Initial Assessment (AASLD 2010)
1. Diagnosis
   a. Give structured questionnaire if concern for abuse of excess alcohol intake (i.e., CAGE, AUDIT)
      i. CAGE: Four questions (cutting down, annoyance by criticism, guilty feelings, and eye-openers); 2+ positive responses predict alcohol abuse[4]
      ii. AUDIT: Ten questions; positive screen is score ≥8 for men <60 years old, ≥4 for women, adolescents, or men >60 years old[5]
   b. Perform lab tests to exclude other etiologies
   c. Evaluate for end-organ damage
   d. Evaluate risk of poor outcome with Maddrey discriminant function (MDF), or serial calculations with MELD score

Acute Medical Management (AASLD 2010)
1. If MDF ≥32, give prednisolone 40 mg/day ×28 days
2. If contraindication to steroids, give pentoxifylline orally 400 mg TID ×4 weeks
3. Give enteral nutritional therapy to those with severe nutritional deficiencies

Interventions (AASLD 2010)
1. Liver biopsy
   a. For severe AH and considering medical treatment or if diagnosis uncertain

Management After Stabilization (AASLD 2010)
1. Encourage strict abstinence
2. Prescribe naltrexone or acamprosate in conjunction with counseling to decrease likelihood of relapse
3. Refer for liver transplant

Source:
1. AASLD 2010. O'Shea R, Dasarathy S, et al. AASLD practice guidelines: alcoholic liver disease. Hepatology. 2010 Jan;51(1). [https://www.aasld.org/sites/default/files/guideline_documents/AlcoholicLiverDisease1-2010.pdf]

CLOSTRIDIUM DIFFICILE INFECTION

Initial Assessment
1. Diagnosis of *C. difficile* (IDSA 2010, ACG 2013)
   a. Test only unformed stool, unless ileus is suspected

---

[4]Ewing, JA. Detecting alcoholism: the CAGE questionnaire. JAMA. 1984;252:1905–1907.
[5]AUDIT – The Alcohol Use Disorders Identification Test: guidelines for use in primary care (second edition), 2001. World Health Organization. http://whqlibdoc.who.int/hq/2001/WHO_MSD_MSB_01.6a.pdf?ua=1

    b. Use PCR for diagnosis

        i. IDSA: Consider two-step analysis: EIA screening with confirmatory cell toxicity assay or toxin culture

        ii. ACG: Two- or three-step testing regimens have lower sensitivity than PCR

    c. ACG: Consider CT abdomen + pelvis for complicated CDI

    d. ACG: Test for CDI when clinically suspected and in those with IBD flare, pregnant, or periparturient with diarrhea

Acute Medical Management (IDSA 2010, ACG 2013)

1. Discontinue offending antibiotic if applicable
2. Avoid anti-peristaltic agents
3. Treat empirically if suspicion is high, even without positive test
4. See Table 5-1 for treatment recommendations

Interventions (IDSA 2010)

1. Consider subtotal colectomy sparing rectum for severely ill patients with serum lactate >5 mmol/L, WBC >50k cells/microliter, hypotension requiring vasopressors, severe sepsis, mental status change, or failure to improve on medical therapy after 5 days

Management After Stabilization (IDSA 2010, ACG 2013)

1. Do not give probiotics for prevention of *C. difficile* infection
2. Consider IVIG in patients with hypogammaglobulinemia
3. ACG: Maintain contact precautions, with hand hygiene and barrier precautions, at least until resolution of the diarrhea
4. ACG: Do not repeat testing or test for cure

Sources:

1. IDSA 2010. Cohen S, Gerding D, et al. SHEA-IDSA Guideline 2010: Clinical practice guidelines for *Clostridium difficile* infection in adults: 2010 update by the Society for Healthcare Epidemiology of America (SHEA) and the Infectious Diseases Society of America (IDSA). Infect Control Hosp Epidemiol. 2010 May;31(3). [https://www.ncbi.nlm.nih.gov/pubmed/20307191]
2. ACG 2013. Surawicz C, Brandt L, et al. Guidelines for the diagnosis, treatment, and prevention of *Clostridium difficile* infections. Am J Gastroenterol. 2013 Apr;108. [https://www.ncbi.nlm.nih.gov/pubmed/23439232]

INFECTIOUS DIARRHEA

Initial Assessment (IDSA 2001)

1. Perform a workup if profuse dehydrating, bloody, or febrile diarrhea; or if patient is infant, elderly, or immunocompromised
2. Take a history including travel history; day care status; ingestion of raw/undercooked meat, seafood, or milk; ill contacts; sexual contacts; medications; medical history

TABLE 5-1

CLOSTRIDIUM DIFFICILE DIAGNOSIS AND TREATMENT BY SOCIETY

Severity	Society	Criteria	Treatment
Mild-to-moderate	ACG	Diarrhea	Metronidazole 500 mg PO QID ×10 days, preferred over vancomycin 125 mg PO QID ×10 days
	IDSA	Diarrhea	Metronidazole[1] 500 mg PO QID ×10–14 days
Severe	ACG	Albumin <3 g/dL + ≥15k WBC or abdominal tenderness	Vancomycin 125 mg PO QID ×10 days
	IDSA	WBC >15k or serum creatinine >1.5× baseline	Vancomycin 125 mg PO QID ×10–14 days
Severe complicated	ACG	Any of the following: ICU admission, hypotension, fever ≥38.5°C, Ileus/distension, mental status change, WBC ≥35k or <2k, serum lactate >2.2 mmol/L, end-organ failure	Vancomycin 500 mg PO QID + metronidazole 500 mg IV q8 hours + vancomycin PR 500 mg in 500 mL saline enema QID
	IDSA	Hypotension/shock, ileus, megacolon	Vancomycin 500 mg QID (PO or NG tube) + metronidazole 500 mg q8 hours IV ± PR[2] vancomycin (if ileus)
Recurrent	ACG	Recurrent CDI within 8 weeks after finishing therapy	Repeat metronidazole or vancomycin pulse regimen; fecal transplant for third recurrence
	IDSA	Second recurrence	Vancomycin tapered and/or pulsed

[1]Avoid prolonged metronidazole use given risk of cumulative neurotoxicity.
[2]PR vancomycin: 500 mg in 100 mL NS q6 hours as retention enema.
Source: Adapted from ACG 2013 and IDSA 2010.

3. Order fecal studies, selectively based on history
   a. Community-acquired or traveler's diarrhea: Test for *Salmonella, Shigella, Campylobacter, Escherichia coli* O157:H7 (include testing for Shiga toxin if blood in stool), and *C. difficile*[6]
   b. Nosocomial diarrhea[7]: Test for *C. difficile*
   c. Persistent diarrhea[8]: Test for parasites (*Giardia, Cryptosporidium, Cyclospora, Isospora belli*); screen for inflammation with fecal lactoferrin testing or fecal leukocytes[9]; if HIV positive test for *Microsporidia, M. avium* complex, and panel A
   d. Seafood or seacoast exposure: Culture for *Vibrio*

Acute Medical Management (IDSA 2001)

1. Rehydrate, orally if possible
2. Treat traveler's diarrhea, shigellosis, or campylobacter
   a. Traveler's diarrhea
      i. Treat empirically with quinolone or trimethoprim-sulfamethoxazole
      ii. Tailor treatment to culture result if culture sent
   b. Nosocomial diarrhea
      i. Discontinue antimicrobials if possible
      ii. Consider metronidazole if illness worsens or persists
   c. Persistent diarrhea
      i. Await test results and tailor therapy accordingly
3. Avoid antimotility agents if diarrhea is bloody or if proven infection with Shiga toxin-producing *E. coli*

Source:

1. IDSA 2001: Guerrant RL, Van Gilder T, Steiner T, et al. Practice guidelines for the management of infectious diarrhea. 2001;32:331–350. [https://www.ncbi.nlm.nih.gov/pubmed/11170940]

ACUTE PANCREATITIS

Initial Assessment (ACG 2013)

1. Diagnose when two of the following present:
   a. Abdominal pain
   b. Serum amylase and/or lipase >3× upper limit of normal
   c. Suggestive imaging

---

[6] Approximately 5% of stool cultures yield a pathogen.
[7] Nosocomial: Onset after >3 days in hospital (stool cultures in first 3 days of hospitalization have very low yield).
[8] Persistent: Duration >7 days, especially if immunocompromised.
[9] If positive lactoferrin or leukocytes without an obvious infectious etiology, workup for inflammatory bowel disease.

2. Do not obtain CT or MRI unless diagnosis is unclear or no improvement within 48–72 hours
3. Obtain transabdominal ultrasound
4. Obtain serum triglyceride[10] if no history of EtOH or evidence of gallstones
5. Consider pancreatic tumor in those >40 years old or genetic testing in those <30 years old if no other cause identified and family history of pancreatic disease
6. Assess hemodynamic status
7. Treat patients with organ failure in the ICU

Acute Medical Management (ACG 2013)

1. Fluids
   a. 250–500 mL/h isotonic crystalloid[11] if no cardiac or renal contraindications
   b. Most beneficial for first 12–24 hours
   c. More rapid infusion if severe volume depletion (hypotension, tachycardia)
   d. Reassess fluid requirements frequently[12] with goal of decreasing blood urea nitrogen
2. Antibiotics (carbapenems, quinolones, or metronidazole)
   a. Give for infected necrosis or extrapancreatic infection (i.e., cholangitis, catheter-acquired infection, bacteremia, UTIs, pneumonias)
   b. Do not routinely use antifungals
   c. Do not give prophylactic antibiotics, including in sterile necrosis

Interventions (ACG 2013)

1. ERCP
   a. Perform within 24 hours if also has acute cholangitis
   b. Do not perform if patient lacks ongoing biliary obstruction
   c. Give post-procedure NSAID suppositories (i.e., 100 mg diclofenac) for high-risk patients without pancreatic duct stents
2. MRCP: If concern for choledocholithiasis without cholangitis or jaundice, perform MRCP or EUS over ERCP
3. Cholecystectomy: Perform prior to discharge[13] if cholelithiasis is present
4. Resection
   a. Infected necrosis
      i. If symptomatic, consider minimally invasive methods of necrosectomy over open debridement
      ii. If stable, wait >4 weeks to allow liquefication of contents and development of fibrous wall

---

[10]Triglycerides >1000 mg/dL suggest hypertriglyceridemia-induced pancreatitis.
[11]Lactated Ringer solution may be preferred.
[12]Reassess within 6 hours of admission and for next 24–48 hours.
[13]If necrotizing, defer until active inflammation subsides and fluid collection resolves/stabilizes.

b. Pancreatic pseudocyst, pancreatic necrosis, extrapancreatic necrosis: Do not perform surgery regardless of size, location, extension

5. CT-guided FNA (for Gram stain and culture)
   a. If concern for infected necrosis
   b. To aid in antibiotic selection
   c. Consider repeating every 5–7 days if culture negative and clinically indicated

Management After Stabilization

1. Nutrition
   a. For mild cases (no nausea or vomiting, resolved abdominal pain), give oral feeds immediately with low-fat solid diet
   b. For severe cases, provide enteral nutrition via nasogastric or nasojejunal delivery
   c. Avoid parenteral nutrition if possible

Source:

1. ACG 2013: Tenner S, Baillie J, DeWitt J, et al. American College of Gastroenterology guideline: management of acute pancreatitis. Am J Gastroenterol. 2013 July 30. doi:10.1038/ajg.2013.218. [http://gi.org/guideline/acute-pancreatitis/]

ACUTE LIVER FAILURE

Initial Assessment (AASLD 2011)

1. Evaluate for toxic ingestion by obtaining history regarding ingestion, amount, and timing of last dose up to 1-year prior
2. Exclude Wilson's disease[14]
3. If history of cancer or massive hepatosplenomegaly obtain imaging and liver biopsy for further evaluation
4. CT head if encephalopathic, to rule out other causes
   a. Grades of encephalopathy
      i. I: Change in behavior with only minimal change in consciousness
      ii. II: Disorientation, drowsy, inappropriate behavior, ±asterixis
      iii. III: Confused, drowsy but arousable to voice, incoherent speech
      iv. IV: Comatose, unresponsive, and decorticate/decerebrate posture

Acute Medical Management (AASLD 2011)

1. Admit, preferably to ICU
2. Suspected acetaminophen overdose[15]

---

[14]Obtain ceruloplasmin, serum, and urinary copper levels, slit lamp examination, hepatic copper levels (when liver biopsy feasible), and total bilirubin/alkaline phosphatase ratio.
[15]Suspected by acetaminophen toxicity nomogram, elevated aminotransferase, and low bilirubin without hypotension or shock.

a. Activated charcoal, if ingestion within 4 hours of presentation

b. N-acetylcysteine (140 mg/kg PO or diluted to 5% solution via NG tube, followed by 70 mg/kg q4 hours ×17 doses); give as early as possible, beneficial within first 48 hours

    i. Acetaminophen overdose

    ii. Elevated serum acetaminophen

    iii. Serum aminotransferase increasing or suggestive of acetaminophen overdose

3. Suspected mushroom poisoning: N-acetylcysteine (as above) and penicillin G (300,000–1 million units/kg/day)

4. Drug-induced liver injury: N-acetylcysteine (as above)

5. Herpes or varicella-induced hepatitis: Acyclovir 5–10 mg/kg IV q8 hours

6. Acute hepatitis B infection: Lamivudine (or another nucleoside analogue)

7. Autoimmune hepatitis: If coagulopathy and mild hepatic encephalopathy, give prednisone 40–60 mg/day

8. If coagulopathy present,[16] give vitamin K (5–10 mg subcutaneously)

9. Treating/preventing CNS complications

a. Encephalopathy: Lactulose

b. Intracranial hypertension: Mannitol (0.5–1 g/kg)

    i. Consider therapeutic hypothermia if refractory to mannitol as a bridge to transplant

c. If high risk for cerebral edema,[17] give hypertonic saline (goal serum Na level 145–155 mEq/L)

d. If patient has seizures, give antiepileptic drugs (phenytoin, benzodiazepines)

e. Therapeutic hypothermia

10. GI prophylaxis

a. Give H2 blockers or PPI to patients in the ICU

b. Use sucralfate as a second-line agent

11. Supportive care

a. Provide support with viral hepatitis A and E (no virus-specific treatment effective)

b. Provide cardiovascular support in ischemic injury and acute liver failure

c. Give maintenance fluids ± bolus with normal saline, or vasopressors for refractory cases (norepinephrine preferred over vasopressin)[18]

    i. Goal MAP ≥75 mmHg and CPP 60–80 mmHg

d. Closely monitor electrolytes and correct as appropriate

---

[16]Consensus guideline.

[17]Serum ammonia >150 μM, hepatic encephalopathy grade III or IV, acute renal failure, or pressor requirements.

[18]Assess volume status with volume challenges, not pulmonary artery catheterization.

Interventions (AASLD 2011)

1. Liver biopsy
   a. If suspected autoimmune hepatitis but negative autoantibodies
   b. To evaluate for malignancy
   c. If diagnosis is elusive
2. Pregnancy: Expeditious delivery if fatty liver of pregnancy or HELLP
3. Intubation for high-grade (III or IV) hepatic encephalopathy
4. Intracranial pressure monitoring[19] if high-grade hepatic encephalopathy
5. Dialysis: If required, continuous preferred over intermittent

Management After Stabilization (AASLD 2011)

1. Discontinue offending agent, if applicable
2. Transplant referral if worsening hepatic function in following cases[20]:
   a. Acetaminophen toxicity (refer early)
   b. Wilson's disease
   c. Autoimmune hepatitis
   d. Acute fatty liver of pregnancy/HELLP without prompt hepatic recovery following delivery
   e. Hepatic vein thrombosis with acute hepatic failure (excluding underlying malignancy)
   f. Mushroom poisoning (often only lifesaving option)
   g. Herpes zoster or varicella zoster infection
   h. High likelihood of death
3. Monitor for infection
   a. Perform serial blood cultures (fungal and bacterial), urine analysis, and chest radiography
4. Coagulopathy management
   a. Transfuse only in setting of thrombocytopenia, prolonged prothrombin time and hemorrhage, or prior to invasive procedure

Source:

1. AASLD 2011: Lee W, Larson A, Stravitz R. AASLD Position Paper: The management of acute liver failure: Update 2011. Hepatology. 2011;55(3):965. [https://www.aasld.org/content/acute-liver-failure-management]

INFLAMMATORY BOWEL DISEASE

Initial Assessment (NICE 2012, NICE 2016)

1. Ulcerative colitis 2016
   a. See Table 5-2 for severity scale

---

[19]Frequent (hourly) neurovascular checks are an alternative where ICP is unavailable.
[20]Do not rely entirely on current scoring systems; they do not adequately predict prognosis.

TABLE 5-2

TRUELOVE AND WITTS' SEVERITY INDEX FOR ULCERATIVE COLITIS			
Symptoms	**Mild**	**Severe**	**Fulminant**
Stools per day	<4	4–6	≥6 + one criteria below (except blood in stool)
Blood in stool	Minimal	Between mild and severe	Gross blood
Temperature >37.8°C	No	No	Yes
Pulse >90 bpm	No	No	Yes
Anemia	No	No	Yes
ESR >30	No	No	Yes

Source: NICE 2016; Table 1.

2. Crohn's disease 2012
    a. Severe active Crohn's disease: Poor overall health and one of the
       following:
        i. Weight loss
        ii. Fever
        iii. Abdominal pain
        iv. Diarrhea

Acute Medical Management to Induce Remission

1. Aminosalicylate
    a. Ulcerative colitis (NICE 2016)
        i. Give for mild or moderate disease
            1. For proctitis/proctosigmoiditis: Give topical (suppository or
               enema) ± oral rather than oral alone
            2. For first presentation/inflammatory exacerbation of left sided/
               extensive UC: High-dose induction of oral aminosalicylate ±
               topical aminosalicylate or oral beclometasone dipropionate
            3. If aminosalicylates not tolerated or contraindicated, give oral
               prednisone instead
2. Corticosteroids
    a. Ulcerative colitis (NICE 2016)
        i. Give for acute severe UC
        ii. If proctitis/proctosigmoiditis with mild or moderate first presentation
            1. Give topical or oral dosing as second-line to aminosalicylate;
               if inadequate response to oral prednisone after 2–4 weeks, add
               tacrolimus to oral prednisolone

    2. Give oral prednisolone in addition to aminosalicylates if no improvement/worsen within 4 weeks

    3. Stop beclometasone diproprionate if adding oral prednisolone

  b. Crohn's disease (NICE 2012)

    i. Give for first presentation or single exacerbation within 12-month period (prednisolone, methylprednisolone, IV hydrocortisone)[21]

    ii. Budesonide is a second-line agent and 5-aminosalicylate is a third-line agent for mild or moderate flares, though they likely have fewer side effects than glucocorticoids

3. IV ciclosporin

  a. Ulcerative colitis (NICE 2016)

    i. Give for acute severe UC if[22]

      1. Minimal/no improvement within 72 hours after starting IV steroids

      2. Worsening symptoms despite IV steroids

      3. Contraindication to IV steroids

      4. Infliximab is an alternative

4. Azathioprine/Mercaptopurine[23]

  a. Crohn's disease (NICE 2012)

    i. Give in conjunction with glucocorticoids[24] or budesonide therapy if ≥2 exacerbations within 12-month period

    ii. Assess thiopurine methyltransferase level to ensure not very low or absent, and consider reduced dosing if low

    iii. Methotrexate is an alternative

5. Infliximab/Adalimumab[25]

  a. Crohn's disease (NICE 2012)

    i. Give for severe flare (as monotherapy or with immunosuppressant) if no response to immunosuppressants ± corticosteroids

    ii. Continue for 12 months or treatment failure (i.e., surgery)

    iii. Infliximab: For active fistulizing Crohn's not responsive to antibiotics, drainage, and immunosuppressants

Interventions

1. Surgical resection

  a. Ulcerative colitis (NICE 2016)

    i. Higher likelihood of requiring surgery if >8 stools/day, fever, tachycardia, dilated colon on radiography, or abnormal labs (low albumin, anemic, elevated platelets, or CRP >45 mg/L)

---

[21] In severe presentations, use steroids alone.
[22] Surgery is a reasonable alternative to starting ciclosporin.
[23] Monitor side effects, including neutropenia.
[24] Glucocorticoid dosing cannot be tapered.
[25] Should be given by experienced clinicians only.

    b. Crohn's disease (NICE 2012)
        i. Consider early surgery for disease limited to distal ileum
2. Balloon dilatation
    a. Crohn's disease (NICE 2012)
        i. Single stricture accessible by colonoscopy, after optimizing medical treatment

Management for Maintaining Remission/Maintenance

1. Aminosalicylates (once-daily dosing)
    a. Ulcerative colitis (NICE 2016)
        i. After mild or moderate flare of proctitis/proctosigmoiditis
            1. Topical aminosalicylate (daily or intermittent) or oral aminosalicylate + topical aminosalicylate preferred over oral aminosalicylate alone
        ii. After mild or moderate flare of left sided or extensive UC
            1. Low-dose oral therapy
        iii. After surgery
        iv. As second-line for severe flare
    b. Crohn's disease (NICE 2012)
        i. After surgery
2. Azathioprine/Mercaptopurine
    a. Ulcerative colitis (NICE 2016)
        i. After severe flare
        ii. After 2+ flares within 12 months requiring systemic steroid treatment
        iii. Unable to achieve remission with aminosalicylates
    b. Crohn's disease (NICE 2012)
        i. Previously naïve to these medicines
        ii. After ≥2 resections
        iii. Previous complicated/debilitating disease (i.e., abscesses, fistulas)
        iv. If used in conjunction with IV steroids to induce remission
3. Methotrexate for maintenance
    a. Crohn's disease (NICE 2012)
        i. Continue if used to induce remission
        ii. Intolerant of or contraindication to mercaptopurine/azathioprine maintenance

Sources:

1. NICE 2012: Crohn's disease: management. National Institute for Health and Care Excellence. 2012 October 10. [https://www.nice.org.uk/Guidance/CG152]
2. NICE 2016: Ulcerative colitis: management. National Institute for Health and Care Excellence. 2016 June 26. [https://www.nice.org.uk/Guidance/CG166]

BOWEL PREPARATION FOR COLONOSCOPY

ASGE 2015

1. Use a split-dose regimen (same-day ok for afternoon procedures) with a portion taken within 3–8 hours of the procedure; individualize to patient and physician needs, considering clinical condition and potential adverse effects of preparation; commercially available preparations include:
   a. Polyethylene glycol with electrolytes (brand: GoLYTELY)
      i. Total amount/single dose: 4 L
      ii. Split dose: 2–3 L day before; 1–2 L day of colonoscopy
   b. Sulfate-free polyethylene glycol with electrolytes (brand: NuLYTELY)
      i. Total amount/single dose: 4 L
      ii. Split dose: 2–3 L day before; 1–2 L day of
   c. Polyethylene glycol 3350 with sports drink (brand: MiraLAX)
      i. Total amount/single dose: 238 g PEG-3350 in 2 L sports drink
      ii. Split dose: 1 L day before; 1 L day of
   d. Oral sodium sulfate
      i. Total amount/single dose: 12 oz with 2.5 L water
      ii. Split dose: 6 oz OSS in 10 oz water + 32 oz water the day before; 6 oz OSS in 10 oz water + 32 oz water the day of
   e. Magnesium citrate
      i. Total amount/single dose: 20–30 oz with 2 L water
      ii. Split dose: 1–1.5 10 oz bottles day before; 1–1.5 10 oz bottles day of
   f. Sodium phosphate tablets
      i. Total amount/single dose: 32 tablets with 2 L water
      ii. Split dose: 20 tablets day before; 12 tablets day of
2. Avoid sodium phosphate and magnesium citrate preparations in elderly patients or patients with renal disease
3. Avoid metoclopramide as an adjunct

Source:

1. ASGE 2015: Saltzman JR, Cash BD, Pasha SF, et al. Bowel preparation before colonoscopy. Gastrointest Endosc. 2015;81:781–794. [http://www.giejournal.org/article/S0016-5107(14)02268-8/abstract]

Infectious Diseases

Neil Jorgensen
Marina Morie

SEPSIS AND SEPTIC SHOCK

Initial Assessment
1. Definitions (SCC 2016)
   a. Sepsis: "Life-threatening organ dysfunction caused by dysregulated host response to infection"
   b. Septic shock: "Subset of sepsis with circulatory and cellular/metabolic dysfunction associated with higher risk of mortality"
2. Diagnosis of sepsis
   a. SSC 2016, NICE 2016: No diagnostic test to define sepsis; clinical diagnosis; treat if suspected or at risk of having sepsis

Sepsis-3 2016: Clinical Criteria for Sepsis: Infection Plus Two or More Points from SOFA Score (See Table 6-1) If Not in ICU, May Use qSOFA Score (Easier Than SOFA)

1. Diagnosis of septic shock
   a. Sepsis-3 2016: Despite adequate fluid resuscitation
      i. Vasopressors required to maintain MAP ≥65 mmHg, AND
      ii. Serum lactate >2 mmol/L
   b. NICE 2016: Infection + fever/feeling unwell, likely source of infection + clinical indicators (behavior/circulation/respiration) + risk factors for sepsis[1] → Stratify risk of severe illness[2]

Acute Medical Management
1. Initial resuscitation
   a. SCC 2016
      i. Give at least 30 mL/kg of IV crystalloid (LR, NS) within 3 hours

[1]Risk factors for sepsis: Age ≥75 years or <1 year, frail with comorbidities, trauma/surgery/invasive procedure within last 6 weeks, impaired immunity, indwelling lines, IV drug use, skin breach (cuts, burns, infection, blisters), pregnant/pregnant in last 6 weeks (particularly if: diabetes or gestational diabetes, c-section/forceps/invasive procedure/retained products, prolonged rupture of membranes, close contact with Group A strep, continued bleeding/offensive vaginal discharge).
[2]NICE 2016 provides detailed guidance on risk assessment, based on behavior, history, breathing, circulation, skin, temperature, and urine, which can be found at http://www.bmj.com/content/354/bmj.i4030/infographic.

TABLE 6-1

SOFA SCORE FOR SEPSIS				

SOFA Score

(*Not recognized by Surviving Sepsis Campaign as diagnostic criterium*):

Screen positive if ≥2 points above baseline of:

Criteria/points	1	2	3	4
Glasgow coma scale	13–14	10–12	6–9	<6
PaO₂:FiO₂ ratio	<400	<300	<200 (w/support)	<100 (w/support)
Systolic blood pressure (vasopressor required)	MAP <70	Dopamine ≤5 or Any dose of dobutamine	Dopamine >5 or epinephrine ≤0.1 or norepinephrine ≤0.1	Dopamine: 15 or epinephrine >0.1 or norepinephrine >0.1
Creatinine or urine output	1.2–1.9	2.0–3.4	3.5–4.9 <500 mL/day	>5.0 <200
Platelets × 10³/mm³	<150	<100	<50	<20
Bilirubin mg/dL	1.2–1.9	2.0–5.9	6.0–11.9	>12.0

qSOFA score				
Screen positive if ≥2 of:				
Altered mentation				
Respiratory rate ≥22 bpm				
Systolic blood pressure ≤100 mmHg				

Source: From Vincent JL, et al. Intensive Care Med. 1996;22(7):707–10; with permission.

   ii. Draw appropriate cultures (two sets of blood cultures – aerobic and anaerobic, and urine/CSF/sputum/abscess if indicated) only if obtaining cultures does not result in substantial delay to starting antimicrobials

   iii. Draw lactate and consider procalcitonin level

 b. NICE 2016

   i. Perform tests including blood cultures, CBC diff, PT/PT, CRP, U/E and creatinine, ABG including glucose and lactate

   ii. Give IV fluids

     1. If lactate ≥2 or SBP <90 give IV crystalloid bolus:

      a. Age >16: 500 mL over ≤15 minutes

      b. Age ≤16: 20 mL/kg over ≤10 minutes

  c. Neonates: Glucose-free crystalloid 10–20 mL/kg over ≤10 minutes

 2. If lactate <2, "consider giving intravenous fluid bolus"

2. Antimicrobials

 a. SSC 2016, NICE 2016: Start IV antimicrobials within 1 hour

 b. SSC 2016

  i. Start empiric broad-spectrum antimicrobials to cover all likely pathogens (bacterial, add fungal or viral coverage if indicated) based on site of infection, local prevalence and resistance, immune defects, age and comorbidities, invasive devices/catheters:

   1. Septic shock: At least two antibiotics of different classes; no specific recommendations; possibilities include a broad-spectrum carbapenem (e.g., meropenem, imipenem/cilastatin, or doripenem) or extended-range penicillin/β-lactamase inhibitor (e.g., piperacillin/tazobactam, ticarcillin/clavulanate) or several third or higher generation cephalosporins

   2. Sepsis without shock or neutropenic sepsis/bacteremia: Do not use routine combination therapy

  ii. For all sepsis

   1. If risk of MDR (multi-drug resistant) gram negatives, e.g., *Pseudomonas, Acinetobacter*, add supplemental gram-negative agent

   2. If risk of methicillin-resistant *Staphylococcus aureus* (MRSA), add anti-MRSA agent, e.g., vancomycin, teicoplanin

   3. If risk of *Legionella*, add macrolide or fluoroquinolone

   4. If risk of *Candida*, add echinocandin (anidulafungin, micafungin, caspofungin); in less ill, echinocandin-intolerant, or non-colonized patients, add a triazole or liposomal amphotericin B

 c. NICE 2016

  i. If meningococcus suspected, use ceftriaxone

  ii. If the source or the history of resistant infections is clear, use local antibiotic guidance

  iii. If source unclear and no history of previous infection/colonization with resistant microbes:

   1. Age ≥18: Use local antibiotic guidelines

   2. Age ≤17: If no resistance, use ceftriaxone 80 mg/kg q24 hours up to 4 g/day

   3. Age <3 months: Ceftriaxone + *Listeria* coverage, e.g., ampicillin

   4. Neonates ≤72 hours: Benzylpenicillin + gentamicin

   5. Neonates from community ≤40 weeks gestational age or received IV calcium: Cefotaxime 50 mg/kg q6–12 hours

   6. Neonates from community >40 weeks gestational age: Ceftriaxone 50 mg/kg q6–12 hours

3. Source control (SCC 2016, NICE 2016)
   a. Identify as rapidly as possible any anatomic source of infection:
      i. Sources more readily to control include intra-abdominal abscesses, GI perforation/ischemia, cholangitis, cholecystitis, urinary obstruction/abscess, soft tissue infection/necrosis, empyema, septic arthritis, other deep space infection, implanted device infection
      ii. Promptly remove intravascular access devices that are possible source of sepsis, after other vascular access established
4. Performance improvement (SCC 2016)
   a. Hospitals should have a performance improvement program for sepsis, including sepsis screening for acutely ill, high-risk patients
   b. Sepsis management bundles shown to decrease mortality were revised in 2015:
      i. Complete within 3 hours of presentation:
         1. Lactate level
         2. Blood cultures
         3. Broad spectrum antibiotics
         4. 30 mL/kg crystalloid for hypotension or lactate $\geq$4 mmol/L
      ii. Complete within 6 hours of presentation:
         1. Vasopressors to maintain MAP $\geq$65 mmHg for persistent hypotension
         2. If MAP still <65 after fluids, or initial lactate $\geq$4 mmol/L, reassess volume status and document:
            a. Repeat focused exam including vital signs, cardiopulmonary, capillary refill, pulse, and skin
         3. OR two of the following:
            a. CVP
            b. ScvO$_2$
            c. Bedside cardiovascular ultrasound
            d. Dynamic assessment with passive leg raise or fluid challenge (dynamic assessments preferred)

Management After Stabilization

1. De-escalation of antimicrobials (SCC 2016)
   a. Assess daily
   b. Treatment duration of 7–10 days is adequate for most serious bacterial infections
      i. Consider longer courses for slow response, undrainable foci, *S. aureus* infection, some fungal and viral infections, immune deficiency/neutropenia
      ii. Consider shorter courses after control of abdominal, urinary source, pyelonephritis with rapid clinical resolution
      iii. Procalcitonin level (see Table 3-3)

      1. Use to shorten duration of antibiotics

      2. Use to stop antibiotics if low level and subsequent evidence of sepsis is weak

   iv. Narrow antibiotics base on culture results or clinical improvement

   v. Stop antibiotics if there is no evidence of infection and evidence of other severe inflammatory state (e.g., burn, pancreatitis)

Sources:

1. Sepsis-3
   a. Shankar-Hari M, Phillips GS, Levy ML, et al. Developing a new definition and assessing new clinical criteria for septic shock for the third international consensus definitions for sepsis and septic shock (Sepsis-3). JAMA. 2016;315:775–787. [https://www.ncbi.nlm.nih.gov/pubmed/26903336]
   b. Singer M, et al. The third international consensus definitions for sepsis and septic shock (Sepsis-3). JAMA. 2016;315(8):801–810. [https://www.ncbi.nlm.nih.gov/pubmed/26903338]
   c. Seymour CW, Liu VX, Iwashyna TJ, et al. Assessment of clinical criteria for sepsis for the third international consensus definitions for sepsis and septic shock (Sepsis-3). JAMA. 2016;315:762–774. [https://www.ncbi.nlm.nih.gov/pubmed/26903335]
2. SSC 2016
   a. Rhodes A, Evans LE, Alhazzani W, et al. Surviving sepsis campaign: international guidelines for the management of sepsis and septic shock: 2016. Crit Care Med. 2017;45:486–552. [http://survivingsepsis.org/SiteCollectionDocuments/SSC-Statements-Sepsis-Definitions-3-2016.pdf]
3. NICE 2016
   a. National Institute for Health and Care Excellence. Sepsis: recognition, diagnosis and early management (NICE guideline 51). 2016. [http://www.nice.org.uk/guidance/ng51]
4. Sepsis Trust. Clinical toolkits. [http://sepsistrust.org/clinical-toolkit/]

SKIN AND SOFT TISSUE INFECTIONS

Initial Assessment (IDSA 2014)

1. Distinguish between types of infection
   a. Nonpurulent
      i. Cellulitis and erysipelas: Does not include inflammation surrounding collections of pus
      ii. Recurrent cellulitis
      iii. Impetigo and ecthyma
      iv. Necrotizing infections, Fournier gangrene

      v. Clostridial gas gangrene and myonecrosis

      vi. Animal bite-related wounds, human bite wounds

      vii. Surgical site infections

      viii. Other skin infections, e.g., cutaneous anthrax, cat scratch disease/bacillary angiomatosis, erysipeloid, glanders, tularemia

      ix. Infections in patients with cancer, neutropenia, or cellular immunodeficiency[3]

  b. Purulent

    i. Furuncles, carbuncles, abscesses

    ii. Recurrent skin abscesses, pilonidal cysts, hidradenitis suppurativa, foreign material

    iii. Purulent lymph nodes, e.g., bubonic plague

2. Obtain gram stain and culture of pus, exudate, abscesses, and suppurative lymph nodes in most skin and soft tissue infections, except:

  a. Reasonable to forego cultures in typical cases of skin abscess, carbuncles, ecthyma, and impetigo

  b. Pus from inflamed epidermoid cysts

  c. Blood, tissue aspirates, or skin biopsy cultures are unnecessary for typical cellulitis

  d. Swabs of vesicle fluid, erosions, or ulcers may be useful in severe/atypical ecthyma

3. Obtain blood cultures in patients who are immunocompromised or have pyomyositis or necrotizing fasciitis

4. Obtain cultures of blood, tissue aspirates, or skin biopsies from patients with severe systemic features (high fever, hypotension), malignancy, immersion injury, animal bites, neutropenia, and severe cell-mediated immunodeficiency

5. Culture swabs of blisters or ulcer base, or biopsy of lesion if suspected cutaneous anthrax

6. Serology often needed to confirm tularemia, cat scratch disease

7. Get MRI to establish diagnosis of pyomyositis (computed tomography (CT) and ultrasound also useful)

8. Early surgical consult/surgical debridement for suspected necrotizing fasciitis, Fournier gangrene, gas gangrene

9. WSES 2014: MRI, CT, and ultrasound in unstable patients may be useful in diagnosing necrotizing infections

10. Consider dermatology consult for patients with cellular immunodeficiency[3]

---

[3]Cellular immunodeficiency includes lymphoma, lymphocytic leukemia, organ transplant recipients, patients on immunosuppressive drugs such as anti-TNF drugs and certain monoclonal antibodies.

Acute Medical Management (IDSA 2014)

1. Purulent infections
   a. Early incision, drainage, and aspiration of purulent foci is primary treatment
   b. Erythema and induration surrounding abscesses may be contiguous inflammation and not cellulitis, not an indication for systemic antibiotics
   c. Do not perform simple needle aspiration (with ultrasound guidance) of abscesses
   d. Covering incision site with dry dressing is sufficient; packing with gauze has not been shown to improve healing
   e. Antibiotics do not improve cure rates; may modestly reduce time to recurrence, consider in patients with impaired host defenses or systemic signs or symptoms
   f. IDSA MRSA 2011: Cover for MRSA empirically pending culture results, in cellulitis with purulent exudate in absence of abscess or disease with multiple sites, rapid progression, systemic signs/symptoms, immunosuppression, comorbidities, very young/elderly, septic phlebitis, unresponsive to I&D, abscess difficult to drain, e.g., in face, hand, genitalia
   g. WSES 2014: Cover MRSA in infections not responding to β-lactam therapy within 48–72 hours

2. Impetigo and ecthyma
   a. Give systemic antibiotics if numerous lesions or during outbreaks of poststreptococcal glomerulonephritis
   b. If *S. aureus involved*, it is usually MSSA; if MRSA suspected[4] or confirmed, use doxycycline, clindamycin, or SMX-TMP

3. Cellulitis
   a. Elevate area affected and treat edema or underlying cutaneous disorders
   b. Lower extremity infections: Examine and treat any intertriginous and web space disease of toes, e.g., tinea pedis
   c. Hospitalize patients with systemic inflammatory response syndrome (SIRS),[5] altered mental status, hemodynamic instability, concern for deeper or necrotizing infection, poor adherence to therapy, outpatient treatment failing, or severely immunocompromised patient

4. Recurrent cellulitis: Treat predisposing conditions, e.g., edema, obesity, eczema, venous insufficiency, toe web disease

5. Necrotizing fasciitis, Fournier gangrene, gas gangrene
   a. Urgent surgical exploration and debridement

---

[4]IDSA 2014: Increased risk for MRSA associated with nasal colonization, prior MRSA infection, recent hospitalization, recent antibiotic use. WSES 2014: Children <2 years old, contact sports, injection drug use, men who have sex with men, military personnel, inmates of correctional facilities/residential homes/shelters, vets/pet owners/pig farmers, recent flu-like illness or severe pneumonia, concurrent SSTI, history of MRSA colonization or infection, antibiotic use in last year (especially quinolones or macrolides).

[5]Temperature >38°C or <36°C, tachypnea >24 br/min, tachycardia >90 bpm, or WBC >12,000 or <4000 cells/μL.

  b. For necrotizing infections, repeat exploration/debridement every 24–36 hours until no further debridement needed
6. Pyomyositis: Early drainage of purulent material
7. Antimicrobials
  a. Consider risk for MRSA[4]
  b. Selection: See Table 6-2
  c. Duration of therapy
      i. Impetigo: Oral × 7 days or topical × 5 days
      ii. Ecthyma: Oral × 7 days
      iii. Erysipelas and cellulitis: 5 days
      iv. Recurrent abscess: 5–10 days after I&D
      v. Surgical site infection: 24–48 hours if antibiotics indicated[6]
      vi. Necrotizing fasciitis: Until no further debridement needed, clinical improvement, and afebrile × 48–72 hours
      vii. Pyomyositis: 2–3 weeks
      viii. Dog or cat bites: 3–5 days if asplenic, immunocompromised, liver disease, edema, moderate-to-severe injury, involvement of periosteum or joint
      ix. Cat scratch disease: Azithromycin × 5 days
      x. Bacillary angiomatosis: 2 weeks–2 months
      xi. Erysipeloid: 7–10 days
      xii. Bubonic plague: Probably 10–14 days
      xiii. Tularemia: 7–10 days, 14 days if severe or oral therapy used
      xiv. Fever and neutropenia, initial episode, bacterial infection: 7–14 days
      xv. Fever and neutropenia, persistent or recurrent: Gram-positive bacteria, *Candida*: 2 weeks following clearance of blood stream infection; Aspergillus: 6–12 weeks
      xvi. Cellular immunodeficiency patients: Susceptible to atypical infections such as non-TB mycobacteria, fungi, *Nocardia*, viruses, and parasites that may require prolonged treatment and suppression

Management After Stabilization
1. IDSA 2014
  a. Bite wounds: Avoid primary closure except for face wounds after copious irrigation, debridement, and prophylactic antibiotics
  b. Tetanus toxoid indicated for clean wounds if no vaccination within past 10 years or dirty wounds if no vaccination within past 5 years
  c. Cellulitis: Consider prednisone 40 mg daily for 7 days in nondiabetic adult patients

---

[6]Treat most surgical site infections with suture removal, evacuation of infected material, dressing changes with healing by secondary intention. Antibiotics indicated if erythema and induration >5 cm from wound edge or systemic signs of infection (Temp. >38.5°C, WBC >12,000, pulse >100 bpm).

TABLE 6-2

ANTIBIOTIC SELECTION FOR SKIN AND SOFT TISSUE INFECTIONS

Infection	Antimicrobial Agent	Adult Dose	Pediatric Dose	Comments
Impetigo (Staphylococcus and Streptococcus)	Mupirocin	Topical BID	Topical BID	For limited number of lesions
	Retapamulin	Topical BID	Topical BID	For limited number of lesions
	Dicloxacillin	250 mg QID PO	N/A	
	Cephalexin	250 mg QID PO	25–50 mg/kg/d÷3–4 PO	
	Clindamycin	300–400 mg QID PO	20 mg/kg/d÷3 PO	
	Amoxicillin-clavulanate	875/125 mg BID PO	25 mg/kg/d of amox÷2 PO	
MSSA	Dicloxacillin	500 mg QID PO	25–50 mg/kg/d÷4 PO	PO of choice in adults
	Nafcillin/Oxacillin	1–2 g q4 h IV	100–150 mg/kg/d÷4 IV	IV drug of choice, not for MRSA
	Cefazolin	1 g q8 h IV	50 mg/kg/d÷3 IV	
	Clindamycin	600 mg q8 h IV or	25–40 mg/kg/d÷3 IV or	For penicillin-allergic non-immediate hypersensitivity, less bone marrow suppression than nafcillin
	Cephalexin	300–400 mg QID PO	25–30 mg/kg/d÷3 PO	
	Doxycycline, minocycline	500 mg QID PO	25–50 mg/kg/d÷4 PO	
		100 mg BID PO	Not recommended for Age <8 y	Inducible resistance in MRSA
	Trimethoprim-sulfamethoxazole	1–2 DS tab BID PO	8–12 mg/kg/d of TMP, ÷2 PO or ÷4 IV	For penicillin-allergic, non-immediate hypersensitivity Limited clinical experience Efficacy poorly documented

(Continued)

TABLE 6-2 (Continued)

ANTIBIOTIC SELECTION FOR SKIN AND SOFT TISSUE INFECTIONS

Infection	Antimicrobial Agent	Adult Dose	Pediatric Dose	Comments
MRSA	Trimethoprim-sulfamethoxazole	1–2 DS tab BID PO	8–12 mg/kg/d of TMP, ÷2 PO or ÷4 IV	Limited efficacy data
	Doxycycline, minocycline	100 mg BID PO	Not recommended for Age <8 years	Limited clinical experience
	Clindamycin	350–450 mg QID PO or 600 mg q8 h IV	30–40 mg/kg/d÷3 PO or 25–40 mg/kg/d÷3 IV	Inducible resistance to MRSA, useful option for children
	Vancomycin	30 mg/kg/d÷2 IV		
	Linezolid	600 mg q12 h IV or 600 mg BID PO		IV drug of choice
	Daptomycin	4 mg/kg q24 h IV	40 mg/kg/d÷4 IV	Expensive, limited clinical experience
	Ceftaroline	600 mg BID IV	10 mg/kg q12 h PO or IV for children <12 years	Risk of myopathy
	Teicoplanin LD	12 mg/kg q12 h IV × 3 doses then 6 mg/kg q12 h	N/A	From WSES 2014
	Tigecycline	100 mg IV × 1 then 50 mg q12 IV	N/A	From WSES 2014
Nonpurulent cellulitis (streptococcal skin infections)	Penicillin	2–4 million units q4–6 h IV	60–100,000 U/kg/dose q6 h	Options for patients with severe penicillin allergy: Clindamycin, vancomycin, linezolid, daptomycin, telavancin
	Clindamycin	600–900 mg q8 h IV	10–13 mg/kg/dose q8 h IV	
	Nafcillin	1–2 g q4–6 h IV	50 mg/kg/dose q6 h IV	
	Cefazolin	1 g q8 h IV	33 mg/kg/dose q8 h IV	
	Penicillin VK	250–500 mg q6 h PO	Not specified	
	Cephalexin	500 mg q6 h PO	Not specified	

Surgical site infections (intestinal or genitourinary)	Ticarcillin-clavulanate	3.1 g q6 h IV
	Piperacillin-tazobactam	3.375 mg q6 h or
	Imipenem-cilastatin	4.5 mg q8 h IV
	Meropenem	500 mg q6 h IV
	Ertapenem	1 g q8 h IV
	Ceftriaxone	1 g q24 h IV
	or Ciprofloxacin	1 g q24 h
	or Levofloxacin	400 mg q12 h IV or
	+Metronidazole	750 mg q12 PO
	Ampicillin-sulbactam	750 mg q24 h IV
	+Gentamicin or	+ 500 mg q8 h IV
	tobramycin	3 g q6 h IV
		5 mg/kg q24 h IV
Surgical site infections (axilla or perineum)	Metronidazole	500 mg q8 h IV
	+	+
	Ciprofloxacin	400 mg q8 h IV or
	or	750 mg q12 h PO
	Levofloxacin	or
	or	750 mg q24 h IV/PO
	Ceftriaxone	1 g q24 h IV
Surgical site infections (other trunk or extremity area)	Oxacillin or nafcillin	2 g q6 h IV
	Cefazolin	0.5–1 g q8 h IV
	Cephalexin	500 mg q6 h PO
	SMX-TMP	1 DS tab q6 h PO
	Vancomycin	15 mg/kg q12 h IV

Consider MRSA coverage with vancomycin 15 mg/kg q12 h IV

TABLE 6-2 (Continued)

ANTIBIOTIC SELECTION FOR SKIN AND SOFT TISSUE INFECTIONS

Infection	Antimicrobial Agent	Adult Dose	Pediatric Dose	Comments
Necrotizing infections Multiple bacteria	Piperacillin-tazobactam + vancomycin Imipenem-cilastatin Meropenem Ertapenem Cefotaxime + Metronidazole or Clindamycin	3.37 g q6–8 h IV + 30 mg/kg/d÷2 1 g q6–8 h IV 1 g q8 h IV 1 g q24 h IV 2 g q6 h IV + 500 mg q6 h IV or 600–900 mg q8 h IV	60–75 mg/kg/dose of Pip q6 h IV + 10–13 mg/kg/dose q8 h IV N/A 20 mg/kg/dose q8 h IV 15 mg/kg/dose q12 h IV 50 mg/kg/dose q6 h IV + 7.5 mg/kg/dose q6 h IV or 10–13 mg/kg/dose q8 h IV	Clindamycin or metronidazole + aminoglycoside or fluoroquinolone if penicillin allergic Ertapenem for age 3 months–12 years
Streptococcus	Penicillin + Clindamycin	2–4 million units q4–6 h IV 600–900 mg q8 h IV	60–100,000 U/kg/dose q6 h IV 10–13 mg/kg/dose q8 h IV	Vancomycin, linezolid, quinupristin/dalfopristin, daptomycin are options if penicillin allergic
S. aureus	Nafcillin/Oxacillin Cefazolin Vancomycin Clindamycin	1–2 g q4 h IV 1 g q8 h IV 30 mg/kg/d÷2 IV 600–900 mg q8 h IV	50 mg/kg/dose q6 h IV 33 mg/kg/dose q8 h IV 15 mg/kg/dose q6 h 10–13 mg/kg/dose q8 h IV	Vancomycin, linezolid, quinupristin/dalfopristin, daptomycin are options if penicillin allergic Use vancomycin for resistant strains Inducible resistance in MRSA

Organism	Antibiotic	Adult Dose	Pediatric Dose
Clostridium	Clindamycin + Penicillin	600–900 mg q8 h IV 2–4 million units q4–6 h IV	10–13 mg/kg/dose q8 h IV 60–100,000 U/kg/dose q6 h IV
Aeromonas hydrophila	Doxycycline + Ciprofloxacin or Ceftriaxone	100 mg q12 h IV 500 mg q12 h IV 1–2 g q24 h IV	Not recommended for pediatric use but may be best option
Vibrio vulnificus	Doxycycline + Ceftriaxone or Cefotaxime	100 mg q12 h IV 1 g QID IV 2 g TID IV	Not recommended for pediatric use but may be best option

Abbreviations: BID, twice daily; QID, 4 times daily; PO, by mouth; mg/kg/d, milligrams per kilogram per day; mg/kg/d ÷ 3–4, milligrams per kilogram per day in 3 to 4 divided doses; amox, amoxicillin; q4h, every 4 hours; IV, intravenous; MSSA, methicillin-sensitive *Staphylococcus aureus*; MRSA, methicillin-resistant *Staphylococcus aureus*; TMP, trimethoprim; TID, 3 times daily; DS, double strength.
Source: IDSA 2014.

2. WSES 2014
  a. De-escalate antibiotics when culture results available
  b. Provide early nutritional support (e.g., 25–30 kcal/kg/day)
3. Prevention
  a. Antibiotic prophylaxis after animal bite-related wounds as above
  b. Recurrent abscesses: Consider *S. aureus* decolonization with intranasal mupirocin BID, daily chlorhexidine washes, and daily decontamination of towels, sheets, and clothes × 5 days
  c. Recurrent cellulitis: If ≥3–4 episodes of cellulitis per year, consider oral penicillin or erythromycin BID × 4–52 weeks or benzathine penicillin IM every 2–4 weeks if predisposing factors persist (e.g., edema, obesity, eczema, venous insufficiency, toe web disease)

Sources:

1. IDSA 2014: Stevens DL, Bisno AL, Chambers HF, et al. Practice guidelines for the diagnosis and management of skin and soft tissue infections: 2014 update by the Infectious Diseases Society of America. Clin Infect Dis. 2014;59(2):e10–e52. [https://www.ncbi.nlm.nih.gov/pubmed/24973422/]
2. IDSA MRSA 2011: Liu C, Bayer A, Cosgrove SE, et al. Clinical practice guidelines by the Infectious Diseases Society of America for the treatment of methicillin-resistant *Staphylococcus aureus* infections in adults and children. Clin Infect Dis. 2011;52(3):e18–e55. [https://www.ncbi.nlm.nih.gov/pubmed/21208910]
3. WSES 2014: Sartelli M, Malangoni MA, May AK, et al. World Society of Emergency Surgery (WSES) guidelines for management of skin and soft tissue infections. World J Emerg Surg. 2014;9(1):57. [https://www.ncbi.nlm.nih.gov/pubmed/25422671]

DIABETIC FOOT INFECTIONS

Initial Assessment (IDSA 2012, IWGDF 2016)

1. Assess and document size, depth, position of diabetic foot ulcers
2. Determine whether infected and classify severity using validated system; use characteristics of wound including erythema, induration, tenderness, warmth and purulence, characteristics of deeper soft tissue, and vital signs
3. See Table 6-3 for severity scoring
4. Assess the affected limb for:
  a. Peripheral arterial disease (PAD) to decide whether revascularization is needed; use ankle-brachial index, especially if pedal pulses diminished[7]

[7]Interpretation of ankle-brachial index (ABI), ratio of systolic blood pressure in ankle: systolic BP in brachial artery.

     b. Venous insufficiency

     c. Biomechanical problems which may predispose to wounds or affect healing (e.g., Charcot joint, hammer toes, bunions, callosities)

     d. Loss of sensation; use a 10 g monofilament fiber

5. IDSA 2012: May use blood tests

     a. Consider complete blood count with differential, erythrocyte sedimentation rate (ESR), C-reactive protein (CRP); may be normal in up to ½ of infected patients but may help predict worse outcomes

     b. Procalcitonin may help detect bacterial infection

6. IDSA 2012, NICE 2015: Debride and clean wound or consult someone with expertise and experience

7. Obtain wound culture, after cleansing and debridement and before starting antibiotics if possible; only if clinically infected

     a. IDSA 2012, IWGDF 2016, NICE 2015: Obtain tissue specimen from base of wound rather than a swab (e.g., curettage or biopsy)

     b. IDSA 2012: Culture aspirates of purulent secretions

     c. NICE 2015: If tissue cannot be obtained, consider a deep swab

8. IDSA 2012, IWGDF 2016, NICE 2015: Obtain an X-ray of the foot to look for osteomyelitis, bony deformity, gas, foreign material

9. Evaluate for presence of osteomyelitis

     a. IDSA 2012, IWGDF 2016: Probe-to-bone (PTB) test; if bone is visible, the wound is infected, or there is gritty bone palpable using sterile blunt metal probe, then osteomyelitis is likely

     b. IWGDF 2016: Elevated inflammatory markers (especially ESR) are suggestive

     c. NICE 2015: Osteomyelitis may be present even with normal inflammatory markers, X-rays, or PTB testing

     d. Imaging (IDSA 2012, IWGDF 2016, NICE 2015)

          i. MRI is preferred imaging if advanced imaging is needed; if not available or feasible, consider CT, SPECT/CT, fluorine-18-fluorodeoxyglusose positron emission tomography (PET), or leukocyte/antigranulocyte scan with bone scan

ABI	Arterial status
>1.30	Poorly compressible vessels, calcification
0.90–1.30	Normal
0.60–0.89	Mild insufficiency
0.40–0.59	Moderate insufficiency
<0.40	Severe insufficiency

TABLE 6-3

DETERMINING DIABETIC FOOT INFECTION SEVERITY

Symptoms/Signs	Wound Classification			
	Uninfected	Mild	Moderate	Severe
Local signs	None	≥2 of: • Erythema >0.5, <2 cm from wound edge • Local swelling/induration • Tenderness or pain • Warmth • Purulent discharge Exclude other inflammatory conditions[1]		Any
Other involvement	None	None	Deeper structures involved (bone, joint, tendon, muscle)	Any
Systemic signs	None	None	None	≥2 of: •Temp. >38 or <36°C •HR >90 beats/min •RR >20/min or $PaCO_2$ <32 mmHg •WBC >12,000 or <4000/mm^3 or >10% bands

[1]Other inflammatory conditions include trauma, gout, acute Charcot, thrombosis, venous stasis.
Source: IDSA 2012; Table 2.

ii. NICE 2015: Consider MRI if osteomyelitis suspected but X-ray negative

iii. IDSA 2012: Consider MRI if plain X-ray negative, wound adequately treated with antibiotics, off-loading, and wound care ≤2 weeks, repeat X-ray still negative, and wound not improving or PTB test positive

e. Bone biopsy (IDSA 2012)

    i. Perform bone biopsy for culture and histology when:

        1. Definitive diagnosis needed to justify early surgery

        2. Tissue or blood cultures are positive for antibiotic-resistant organisms which are likely causes of osteomyelitis

        3. With or without surgical resection when there is progressive bone destruction or ESR/CRP remain elevated despite empiric- or culture-directed therapy

        4. Insertion of orthopedic metal ware is planned

        5. Do not use cultures from soft tissue or sinus tracts

Acute Medical Management

1. Consider nonsurgical management of osteomyelitis when:

    a. Surgical resection would cause unacceptable loss of function

    b. Limb ischemia is not amenable to revascularization and the patient wishes to avoid amputation

    c. Infection involving the forefoot only and minimal soft tissue loss

    d. Risks of surgery outweigh the benefits

2. Antibiotics

    a. General principles (NICE 2015, IWGDF 2016, IDSA 2012)

        i. Do not treat clinically uninfected wounds with antibiotics

        ii. Choose antibiotics based on severity, care setting, patient preferences, clinical situation, medical history, cost, clinical response to previous antibiotics, and microbiology results

        iii. IDSA 2012: Establish guidelines for antibiotics accounting for local patterns of resistance

        iv. IDSA 2012: Start antibiotics as soon as possible, preferably after cultures and samples taken

        v. IDSA 2012: Do not use tigecycline if avoidable

    b. Antibiotic selection (IDSA 2012)

        Source: IDSA 2012; Table 8, p. 151-2.

        i. Table 6-4 gives suggested antibiotics

    c. Duration of antibiotic therapy

        i. NICE 2015, IWGDF 2016

            1. Do treat mild infections for longer than 14 days, 1–2 weeks is usually sufficient

            2. Treat osteomyelitis (if infected bone not resected) for prolonged period, usually 6 weeks

TABLE 6-4

SUGGESTED ANTIBIOTIC SELECTION FOR DIABETIC FOOT INFECTION

Severity/Route	Likely Pathogen	Antibiotic	Comments
Mild/Usually oral	MSSA *Streptococcus*	Dicloxacillin, cephalexin Levofloxacin Amoxicillin-clavulanate Clindamycin	QID, inexpensive Daily, may miss *S. aureus* Includes anaerobic coverage May also be active vs. MRSA, check macrolide sensitivity, consider "D-test"
	MRSA Pending cultures, empirically treat MRSA when: • History of previous MRSA or colonization in past year • Local prevalence of MRSA is high (e.g., 50% of all *S. aureus* isolates for mild, 30% for moderate infection) • Unacceptable risk of treatment failure	Doxycycline, Trimethoprim/Sulfamethoxazole	May miss some *Streptococcus*
Moderate or Severe/Moderate: Start oral or Parenteral Severe: Start parenteral	MSSA *Streptococcus*, Enterobacteriaceae Obligate anaerobes	Levofloxacin Cefoxitin Ceftriaxone Ampicillin–sulbactam Moxifloxacin Ertapenem	Daily, may miss *S. aureus* Anaerobe coverage Once daily Poor coverage of *Pseudomonas* Once daily, broad spectrum, vs. most anaerobes Once daily, broad spectrum, vs. most anaerobes, misses *Pseudomonas*

Switch to oral when infection is responding	Levofloxacin or ciprofloxacin With clindamycin Imipenem–cilastatin Tigecycline	PO and IV both available, uncertain efficacy of clindamycin vs. severe S. aureus infection Very broad-spectrum, not vs. MRSA, restrict use, e.g., when ESBL-producer suspected Covers MRSA, not recommended NICE 2015 and increased mortality warning
MRSA Cover severe infections for MRSA; also cover when evidence of infection or colonization elsewhere, or risk factors noted above	Linezolid Daptomycin Vancomycin	Expensive, increased risk toxicity if >2 weeks Once daily, rhabdomyolysis risk: Monitor CPK Increasing MICs for MRSA
Pseudomonas aeruginosa Usually not a pathogen, consider coverage when there is high local prevalence, warm climate, or frequent exposure to water	Piperacillin–tazobactam	Dose every 6 or 8 hours, also broad spectrum
MRSA, Enterobacteriaceae, Pseudomonas, and anaerobes	Vancomycin + Ceftazidime, Or cefepime, Or piperacillin–tazobactam, Or aztreonam, Or a carbapenem	For very broad-spectrum coverage For empiric coverage of severe infection: Use of ceftazidime, cefepime, or aztreonam May require additional anaerobe coverage

Some of these agents are not FDA approved for treating diabetic or complicated skin and soft tissue infections.

Abbreviations: MSSA, Methicillin-susceptible *Staphylococcus aureus*; QID, 4 times a day; MRSA, methicillin-resistant *Staphylococcus aureus*; PO, by mouth; IV, Intravenous; MICs, minimum inhibitory concentrations.

Source: IDSA 2012; Table 8.

     ii. IDSA 2016

        1. Mild infections, topical or oral, 1–2 weeks

        2. Moderate infections, oral or initial parenteral, 1–3 weeks

        3. Severe, parenteral then switch to oral, 2–4 weeks

        4. Osteomyelitis

           a. No remaining infected tissue: Parenteral or oral, 2–5 days

           b. No remaining infected bone but residual soft tissue: Parenteral or oral, 1–3 weeks

           c. Remaining infected but viable bone: Parenteral then switch to oral, 4–6 weeks

           d. No surgery or remaining dead bone: Parenteral then switch to oral, ≥3 months

           e. Extend therapy if wound remains clinically infected

  3. Wound care

    a. Local treatment (IDSA 2012)

      i. Debride the wound to remove necrotic/nonviable tissue, slough, or foreign material and surrounding callus; sharp debridement is usually preferable

      ii. Do not use topical antimicrobials in uninfected wounds; do not use silver-based dressings in clinically infected wounds

    b. Dressings (IDSA 2012, IWGDF 2016)

      i. Use dressings that produce a moist healing environment and control excess exudation

      ii. No specific type of dressing has been shown to prevent infection or improve outcomes

    c. Off-loading pressure (IDSA 2012)

      i. Remove pressure from a diabetic foot wound; the modality is based on location, presence of PAD, severity of infection, physical/social/psychological characteristics of the patient

      ii. Consider removable or non-removable total contact cast or other off-loading devices

    d. Adjunctive therapies

      i. IDSA 2012

        1. No adjunctive therapy has been shown to help heal most wounds

        2. For selected slow-healing wounds, may consider bioengineered skin equivalents, growth factors, granulocyte colony-stimulating factors, hyperbaric oxygen therapy, or negative pressure therapy

      ii. NICE 2015

        1. Do not offer growth factors or hyperbaric oxygen therapy

    2. For non-healing wounds, consider negative pressure therapy and dermal/skin substitutes

Interventions

1. Get a surgical consult (IDSA 2012, IWGDF 2016)
   a. URGENTLY if there is gas in deep tissues, abscess, compartment syndrome, and necrotizing fasciitis
      i. Other signs requiring urgent surgery:
         1. Evidence of systemic inflammatory response
         2. Exam finding rapid progression, necrosis or gangrene, crepitus, bullae (especially hemorrhagic), new onset anesthesia or loss of neurologic function, pain out of proportion, limb ischemia, extensive soft tissue loss
         3. Imaging shows gas, extensive bony destruction especially midfoot/hindfoot
   b. IDSA 2012: For substantial nonviable tissue, substantial bone or joint involvement
   c. For selected moderate and all severe infections (see Table 6-3 for definitions)
   d. When there is clinical or imaging evidence of ischemia in the affected limb (vascular surgeon)
   e. When osteomyelitis is present and
      i. There is persistent unexplained sepsis
      ii. Patient unable to receive or tolerate appropriate antibiotics
      iii. Progressive bony deterioration while on appropriate therapy
      iv. Bony destruction compromises foot mechanics
      v. Patient wishes to avoid prolonged antibiotics, desire to speed wound healing
      vi. To allow more treatable soft tissue wound/allow closure
      vii. Comorbidities make prolonged antibiotics relatively contraindicated or less effective (e.g., kidney disease)

Management After Stabilization

1. Antibiotic therapy
   a. IDSA 2012, NICE 2015: Narrow therapy when culture and sensitivity results available
   b. IDSA 2012, IWGDF 2016: Switch to oral therapy if appropriate, when the patient is systemically well, the infection is responding, and cultural results are available
   c. IDSA 2012
      i. Continue antibiotics until resolution of clinical infection
      ii. Do not continue antibiotics after infection is clinically resolved, even if wound is not completely healed

2. Nonresponse to treatment (IDSA 2012)
   a. Wounds may take ≥20 weeks to heal; in non-healing wounds, consider failure of:
      i. Adherence to wound care regimen
      ii. Adequate wound debridement
      iii. Adequate dressings
      iv. Adequate off-loading
      v. Identification and treatment of PAD
      vi. Malignancy in lesion (consider biopsy for pathology)
      vii. Identification and treatment of other infection
   b. In persistent or refractory signs of infection, consider failure of:
      i. Identification or treatment of PAD
      ii. Identification of remaining necrotic soft tissue or bone
      iii. Drainage of abscesses
      iv. Adequate debridement of wound
      v. Response to treatment of osteomyelitis
      vi. Identification of untreated pathogen
      vii. Adequate delivery of antibiotics
      viii. Adherence to antibiotic regimen
      ix. Correction of metabolic derangements

Sources:

1. IDSA 2012: Lipsky BA, Berendt AR, Cornia PB, et al. Executive summary: 2012 Infectious Diseases Society of America clinical practice guideline for the diagnosis and treatment of diabetic foot infections. Clin Infect Dis. 2012;54(12):1679–1684. [https://www.ncbi.nlm.nih.gov/pubmed/22619242]
2. IWGDF 2016: Lipsky BA, Aragon-Sanchez J, Diggle M, et al. International Working Group on the Diabetic Foot. IWGDF guidance on the diagnosis and management of foot infections in persons with diabetes. Diabetes Metab Res Rev. 2016;32(Suppl 1):45–74. [https://www.ncbi.nlm.nih.gov/pubmed/26386266]
3. NICE 2015: National Institute for Health and Care Excellence (NICE). Diabetic foot problems: prevention and management. London (UK): National Institute for Health and Care Excellence (NICE); 2015 Aug 26. 47 p. (NICE guideline; no. 19). [https://www.nice.org.uk/guidance/ng19]

INFLUENZA

Diagnosis (IDSA 2009)

1. Who to test for influenza
   a. During influenza season

      i. Immunocompetent patients at high risk for complications of influenza with acute febrile respiratory symptoms within 5 days of illness onset[8]

      ii. Immunocompromised patients with febrile respiratory symptoms at any time in the illness course[9]

      iii. Hospitalized patients with a fever and respiratory symptoms at any time in the illness course

      iv. Elderly/infants/children with fever of unknown source with or without respiratory symptoms at any time in the illness course

      v. Any patient who develops fever and respiratory symptoms after hospital admission at any time in the illness course

  b. Any time of year

      i. Health care personnel, residents, or visitors in an institution with an influenza outbreak with febrile respiratory symptoms within 5 days of illness onset

      ii. Patients linked to an influenza outbreak within 5 days of illness onset

2. Specimen collection for influenza testing

  a. Collect within 5 days after illness onset, especially in older children and adults

      i. Infants/young children: Nasal aspirates and swabs

      ii. Older children/adults: Nasopharyngeal aspirates and swabs

      iii. Oropharyngeal and sputum specimens have a lower yield for detection of human influenza viruses

  b. In immunocompromised patients or patients on mechanical ventilation, consider upper and lower respiratory tract specimens within 5 days after illness onset for influenza testing

  c. Do not use acute phase serum specimens for diagnosis

3. Methods of testing for influenza

  a. Choose a method that can yield a timely result and interpret based on the patient's presentation, sensitivity/specificity of the test, and the present influenza activity in the community

Treatment (IDSA 2009)

1. Who to treat

  a. Patients with lab-confirmed or high suspected influenza virus infection at high risk of developing complications,[10] within 48 hours after symptom onset

---

[8]When the virus is typically being shed.

[9]Immunocompromised patients can shed the virus for weeks to months.

[10]Unvaccinated infants 12–24 months, patients with asthma or other chronic pulmonary disease, hemodynamically significant cardiac disease, immunosuppressive disorders or receiving immunosuppressive therapy, HIV+, sickle cell anemia or other hemoglobinopathies, disease that requires long-term ASA therapy (e.g., rheumatoid arthritis, Kawasaki disease), chronic renal dysfunction, cancer, chronic metabolic disease (e.g., diabetes mellitus), neuromuscular disorders, seizure disorders, or cognitive dysfunction affecting handling of respiratory secretions, BMI >40, American Indians, Alaskan natives, pregnant patients, patients >65 years, and residents of nursing homes/long-term care institutions.

Test	Time to result	Comments
RT-PCR	2 hours	High sensitivity/very high specificity; highly recommended
Immunofluorescence	2–4 hours	Moderate high sensitivity/high specificity; recommended
Direct fluorescent antibody staining	2–4 hours	Detects/distinguishes between influenza A & B and between A/B and other respiratory viruses
Indirect fluorescent antibody staining	2–4 hours	Detects/distinguishes between influenza A & B and between A/B and other respiratory viruses
Rapid influenza diagnostic tests		Low-to-moderate sensitivity/high specificity; recommended
Antigen detection (EIA)	10–20 minutes	Depending on EIA test, can detect influenza A only, detect/distinguish between influenza A & B, or detect but not distinguish influenza A/B
Neuraminidase detection assay	20–30 minutes	Detects but not distinguish between influenza A & B
Viral culture		Moderate-to-high sensitivity/highest specificity; best for confirming screening tests and public health surveillance, not for timely clinical management
Shell vial culture	48–72 hours	
Isolation in cell culture	3–10 days	
Serologic tests		Only in reference laboratories; not useful for timely clinical management

b. Patients requiring hospitalization for lab-confirmed or highly suspected influenza illness, within 48 hours after symptom onset; those who require hospitalization for influenza may benefit from treatment even >48 hours after symptom onset

c. Consider treatment in patients at high risk of complications with illness that is not improving and have a positive influenza test >48 hours after symptom onset

d. Consider treatment in low-risk patients with positive influenza test <48 hours after symptom onset, who wish to shorten their duration or illness and reduce their relatively low risk of complications, or who are in close contact with high-risk patients; approximately 1 day decrease in illness duration

2. Antiviral drug choice
   a. Influenza A
      i. (H1N1): Zanamivir or an adamantane (preferably rimnatadine); do not use oseltamivir
      ii. (H3N2): Olsetamivir or zanamivir; do not use adamantanes
      iii. If no subtyping available, use zanamivir or oseltamivir + rimantadine
   b. Influenza B: Oseltamivir or zanamivir
   c. When oseltamivir resistance is suspected, use IV zanamivir, available on a compassionate use basis from its manufacturer with FDA approval
3. Chemoprophylaxis
   a. Not a substitute for influenza vaccination, the primary tool for prevention
   b. Consider in the following settings:
      i. High-risk patient during the 2 weeks after vaccination (or 6 weeks for children who were not previously vaccinated)[11] when influenza viruses are circulating in the community
      ii. High-risk patients for whom the influenza vaccine is contraindicated[12]
      iii. Unvaccinated adults who are in close contact with patient at high risk for developing influenza complications
   c. Give in the following settings:
      i. All residents, regardless of vaccine status, who live in nursing homes/long-term care institutions that are experiencing influenza outbreaks
      ii. High-risk patients who are not protected due to poor immune response, lack of influenza vaccine, or ineffective vaccine; initiate chemoprophylaxis at the onset of sustained community influenza activity and continue throughout the duration of the influenza season for that community
   d. Duration of chemoprophylaxis
      i. Stop 2 weeks after vaccination for patients in noninstitutional settings (6 weeks for children receiving the influenza vaccine for the first time)
      ii. Continue chemoprophylaxis for 10 days if used in a household after diagnosis of influenza in one family member
      iii. Continue chemoprophylaxis for 14 days or for 7 days after the onset of symptoms in the last person infected (whichever is longer) in the setting of an institutional outbreak
   e. Antiviral selection for chemoprophylaxis is the same as for treatment

---

[11] To allow an adequate immune response to inactivated vaccine.
[12] Anaphylactic hypersensitivity to eggs or other vaccine components, moderate to severe febrile illness, history of Guillain-Barré syndrome within 6 weeks after receipt of a prior influenza vaccination.

Agent	Treatment	Chemoprophylaxis
Neuraminidase inhibitors		
Oseltamivir	75 mg capsule BID ×5 days	75 mg capsule QD
Zanamivir	Two 5 mg inhalations BID	Two 5 mg inhalations QD
Adamantanes		
Rimantadine	200 mg per day, QD or divided BID	200 mg per day, QD or divided BID
Amantadine	200 mg per day, QD or divided BID	200 mg per day, QD or divided BID

Source:

1. IDSA 2009: Harper SA, Bradley JS, Englund JA, et al. Seasonal influenza in adults and children – diagnosis, treatment, chemoprophylaxis, and institutional outbreak management: clinical practice guidelines of the Infectious Diseases Society of America. Clin Infect Dis. 2009;48(8):1003–1032. [https://www.ncbi.nlm.nih.gov/pubmed/19281331]

VERTEBRAL OSTEOMYELITIS

Initial Assessment

1. When to consider the diagnosis of vertebral osteomyelitis (VO) (IDSA 2015, UMHS 2013)
   a. Evaluate a patient for VO if they have new or worsening back or neck pain and suggestive clinical features
   b. IDSA: Evaluate for VO in patient with fever and new neurologic symptoms with or without back pain
2. Clinical features
   a. With new or worsening back or neck pain (IDSA 2015)
      i. Fever
      ii. Elevated ESR or CRP
      iii. Bloodstream infection or infective endocarditis
   b. With new localized back or neck pain (IDSA 2015)
      i. Recent episode (e.g., past 3 months) of *S. aureus* bloodstream infection
   c. Other clinical features (UMHS 2013)
      i. Neurologic symptoms
         1. Limb weakness
         2. Dysesthesia
         3. Radicular pain

       4. Gait disturbance

       5. Bowel/bladder dysfunction

    ii. Symptoms specific to spinal location of VO, e.g.,

       1. Dysphagia with cervical involvement

       2. Autonomic dysregulation with thoracic VO

3. If a patient does not have at least one risk factor for VO, consider alternate diagnosis (UMHS 2013)

  a. Risk factors

    i. Diabetes (most common risk factor)

    ii. IV drug use (IVDU)

    iii. Indwelling vascular device

    iv. Immunosuppression

    v. Malignancy

    vi. Cirrhosis

    vii. Chronic kidney disease

    viii. Alcohol use

    ix. HIV/AIDS

    x. Rheumatoid arthritis

    xi. Spinal trauma history

    xii. Recent spinal procedure

    xiii. Other focus of infection

4. Evaluation (IDSA 2015, UMHS 2013)

  a. Complete neurologic exam

  b. Consult spinal surgeon and infectious disease specialist; sooner if abnormal exam

  c. Blood tests: CBC (complete blood count), ESR, CRP, two sets of blood cultures

    i. UMHS 2013: Also, basic metabolic panel, urine analysis/culture

    ii. IDSA 2015

       1. Blood cultures and serologic tests for *Brucella* if subacute VO and in endemic area

       2. Blood cultures and serologic tests for fungi if at risk[13] for fungal infection

       3. Purified protein derivative (PPD) test or interferon-γ release assay if at risk for tuberculosis (i.e., from endemic area or residential risk)

  d. Imaging (IDSA 2015, UMHS 2013)

    i. Obtain MRI of complete spine (with and without contrast)

    ii. IDSA 2015: If MRI contraindicated or unavailable, get gallium/Tc99 bone scan, CT scan, or PET scan

---

[13] Epidemiologic risk (e.g., blastomycosis, coccidioidomycosis, histoplasmosis areas) or host risk (e.g., immunosuppression, IVDA, indwelling IV catheter).

iii. UMHS 2013: If MRI not possible, get CT myelogram or CT with contrast

e. Biopsy (IDSA 2015)

  i. Perform image-guided aspiration biopsy of affected area if suspected VO, unless

   1. Patient has known bloodstream infection with *S. aureus*, *Staphylococcus lugdunensis*, or *Brucella*

   2. Patient has strongly positive *Brucella* serology

  ii. Send biopsy specimen for

   1. Bacterial culture, aerobic and anaerobic

   2. Pathology (for inflammation, granulomas, malignancy), if adequate tissue obtained

   3. Fungal, mycobacterial, or *Brucella* cultures, if risk based on host, epidemiologic, or imaging appearance

  iii. If initial biopsy is nondiagnostic, or grows organism which is usually skin contaminant (i.e., coagulase negative staphylococci (except *S. lugdunensis*), *Propionibacterium*, diphtheroids), and blood cultures negative, repeat aspiration biopsy

  iv. If initial biopsy nondiagnostic and blood cultures negative

   1. Test further for anaerobes, fungi, *Brucella*, mycobacteria, other difficult-to-grow organisms

   2. Repeat image-guided aspiration biopsy, percutaneous endoscopic discectomy and drainage, or open excisional biopsy

  v. UMHS 2013: If imaging shows VO, arrange for image-guided biopsy within 24 hours

Acute Medical Management

1. Urgent management (IDSA 2015, UMHS 2013)

   a. If neurologic compromise, impending sepsis, or hemodynamically unstable

      i. Urgent surgical consultation and intervention

      ii. Begin empiric antibiotics (see Table 6-5)

   b. UMHS 2013: Neurologic checks every 4 hours while hospitalized

2. Antibiotics (IDSA 2015)

   a. If normal, stable neurologic exam and hemodynamics, hold empiric antibiotics until organism identified (may be up to 1–2 weeks)

   b. If unstable, i.e., septic, in septic shock, sever or progressive neurologic deficits, start empiric antibiotics while obtaining cultures/serologies (IDSA 2015, UMHS 2013)

   c. Specific antibiotic recommendations: See Table 6-6

3. Duration of therapy (IDSA 2015)

   a. Treat most bacterial VO with total of 6 weeks parenteral or highly bioavailable oral antibiotics

TABLE 6-5

EMPIRIC TREATMENT OF VERTEBRAL OSTEOMYELITIS		
UMHS 2013	Preferred[1]	Vancomycin IV + Ceftriaxone 2 g IV q12 h
	For suspected *Pseudomonas*	Vancomycin IV + cefepime 2 g IV q8 h
	For non-anaphylactic penicillin allergy	Vancomycin IV + meropenem 2 g IV q8 h
	For severe penicillin allergy	Vancomycin IV + aztreonam 2 g IV q8 h
	For vancomycin allergy or intolerance	Linezolid 600 mg IV q12 h to replace vancomycin in above regimens
IDSA 2015	General recommendations	Vancomycin + 3rd or 4th generation cephalosporin Vancomycin + ciprofloxacin Vancomycin + cefepime Vancomycin + carbapenem
	Alternative	Daptomycin + quinolone

[1]These doses include treatment of spinal epidural abscess and may be lower for prolonged treatment of VO.
Abbreviations: 2 g, 2 grams; IV, intravenous; q12 h, every 12 hours.
Source: Adapted from UMHS 2013, IDSA 2015.

  b. Treat *Brucella* VO for 3 months
  c. See organism-specific guidelines for treatment of fungal or mycobacterial VO

Management After Stabilization (2015)

1. Monitor ESR and/or CRP after 4 weeks of antibiotics
2. Assess regularly for change in clinical status
3. Determining treatment failure
  a. Not necessarily treatment failure if there is persistent pain, residual neurologic defects, elevated ESR/CRP, or findings on imaging
  b. Suspect treatment failure if:
    i. Unchanged or increasing ESR/CRP after 4 weeks of treatment (patients with 50% reduction in ESR after 4 weeks rarely develop treatment failure)
    ii. Persistent or progressive pain, systemic symptoms of infection
4. If treatment failure suspected
  a. Repeat MRI, attention to paraspinal and epidural soft tissue changes
  b. If clinical or MRI evidence of treatment failure, repeat aspiration or surgical biopsy to test for cultures, histology, and pathology

TABLE 6-6

TREATMENT OF SPECIFIC ORGANISMS IN NATIVE VERTEBRAL OSTEOMYELITIS

Pathogen	Preferred	Alternatives	Notes
Staphylococcus (oxacillin susceptible)	Nafcillin/Oxacillin 1.5–2 g IV q6 h or continuous Cefazolin 1–2 g IV q8 h Ceftriaxone 2 g IV q24 h	Vancomycin 15–20 mg/kg IV q12 h[1] Daptomycin 6–8 mg/kg IV q24 h Linezolid 600 mg PO/IV q12 h Levofloxacin 500–750 mg PO q24 h with rifampin 600 mg PO daily Clindamycin 600–900 mg IV q8 h	
Staphylococcus (oxacillin resistant)	Vancomycin 15–20 mg IV q12 h[1]	Daptomycin 6–8 mg IV q24 h Linezolid 600 mg PO/IV q12 h Levofloxacin 500–750 mg PO q24 h with rifampin 600 mg PO daily	
Enterococcus spp. (penicillin susceptible)	Penicillin G 20–24 million units IV q24 h Continuously or ÷ 6 Ampicillin 12 g IV q24 h continuously or ÷ 6	Vancomycin 15–20 mg IV q12 h[1] Daptomycin 6 mg/kg IV q24 h Linezolid 600 mg PO/IV q12 h	Vancomycin only if penicillin allergic Consider addition of 4–6 weeks of aminoglycoside especially if also have infective endocarditis
Enterococcus spp. (penicillin resistant)	Vancomycin 15–20 mg IV q12 h[1]	Daptomycin 6 mg/kg IV q24 h Linezolid 600 mg PO/IV q12 h	
Pseudomonas aeruginosa	Cefepime 2 g IV q8–12 h Meropenem 1 g IV q8 h Doripenem 500 mg IV q8 h	Ciprofloxacin 750 mg PO q12 Or 400 mg IV q8 h Ceftazidime 2 g IV q8 h Aztreonam 2 g IV q8 h	Aztreonam for severe penicillin allergic or quinolone-resistant strain

Organism			Comments
Enterobacteriaceae	Cefepime 2 g IV q12 h Ertapenem 1 g IV q24 h	Ciprofloxacin 500–750 mg IV q12 h Or 400 mg IV q12 h Moxifloxacin 400 mg PO daily Levofloxacin 500–750 mg PO daily Ciprofloxacin 500–750 mg PO BID Trimethoprim-sulfamethoxazole DS 1–2 tablets PO BID	May need to monitor sulfamethoxazole level
β-hemolytic *Streptococcus*	Penicillin G 20–24 million units IV q24 h Continuously or ÷ 6 Ceftriaxone 2 g IV q24 h	Vancomycin 15–20 mg IV q12 h[1]	Vancomycin only if penicillin allergic
Propionibacterium acnes	Penicillin G 20 million units IV q24 h Continuously or ÷ 6 Ceftriaxone 2 g IV q24 h	Clindamycin 600–900 mg IV q8 h Vancomycin 15–20 mg IV q12 h[1]	Vancomycin only if penicillin allergic
Salmonella spp.	Ciprofloxacin 500 mg PO q12 h Or 400 mg IV q12 h	Ceftriaxone 2 g IV q24 h	Ceftriaxone if isolate nalidixic acid resistant, consider 8-week course
Bacteroides spp., other susceptible anaerobes	Metronidazole 500 mg PO TID-QID		Can be used in initial course
Brucella	Streptomycin then doxycycline Doxycycline + Rifampin		3-month course

[1]Vancomycin may be given with initial loading dose, adjust dose based on renal and hepatic function, monitor serum levels.

Abbreviations: g, grams; IV, Intravenous; PO, oral; q6h, every 6 hours; ÷6, in 6 divided doses; BID, 2 times daily; TID, 3 times daily; QID, 4 times daily.

Source: IDSA 2015; Table 2.

c. If persistent or recurrent bloodstream infection without other source, or worsening pain, consult surgery for debridement with or without stabilization

d. Do not perform surgical debridement for bony imaging findings alone in a patient who is improving clinically (symptoms, physical exam, and inflammatory markers)

Sources:

1. IDSA 2015: Berbari EF, Kanj SS, Kowalski TJ, et al. 2015 Infectious Diseases Society of America (IDSA) clinical practice guidelines for the diagnosis and treatment of native vertebral osteomyelitis in adults. Clin Infect Dis. 2015 Sep 15;61(6):e26–e46. [https://www.ncbi.nlm.nih.gov/pubmed/26229122/]

2. UMHS 2013: University of Michigan Health System. Vertebral osteomyelitis, discitis, and spinal epidural abscess in adults. Ann Arbor (MI): University of Michigan Health System; 2013 Aug. 11 p. [https://www.guideline.gov/summaries/summary/47349]

PROSTHETIC JOINT INFECTIONS

Initial Assessment (IDSA 2013)

1. Consider the diagnosis of prosthetic joint infection (PJI) when there is:
   a. A sinus tract or persistent wound drainage over the prosthetic joint
   b. Acute onset of pain in the prosthesis
   c. Chronically painful prosthesis, especially if never pain-free
   d. Pain and a history of prior problems with wound healing or infection
2. Evaluation for suspected PJI
   a. Laboratory studies
      i. Test for ESR and CRP (AAOS 2010, IDSA 2013)
      ii. Get blood cultures if there is a fever or other condition or infection that would make bloodstream infection more likely (IDSA 2013)
   b. Imaging
      i. Get a plain X-ray (IDSA 2013)
      ii. Do not routinely use other imaging (MRI, CT, scans) (IDSA 2013)
      iii. Nuclear imaging (particularly FDG-PET per 2012 guideline), including also labeled leukocyte imaging (± bone scan/bone marrow imaging), gallium imaging is an option if infection is not established and surgery not planned (AAOS 2010, 2012)
   c. Obtain orthopedic consultation (IDSA 2013)
   d. Arthrocentesis
      i. If medically stable, withhold any antibiotics for 2 weeks, then perform arthrocentesis, unless surgery is planned, if (IDSA 2013)
         1. Suspected infection is acute

2. Suspected infection is chronic and elevated ESR or CRP

3. There is clinical suspicion for PJI

  ii. Knee affected: Aspirate if abnormal ESR and/or CRP (AAOS 2010)

  iii. Hip affected (AAOS 2010): See Table 6-7

  iv. Repeat aspiration of hip or knee if there is discrepancy between likelihood of infection and culture result (AAOS 2010)

e. Synovial fluid analysis

  i. Send aspirated fluid for aerobic and anaerobic culture, synovial fluid white blood cell count (WBC) and differential (AAOS 2010, IDSA 2013)

  ii. Do not use Gram stain results to rule out infection (AAOS 2010)

  iii. Send fluid for a crystal analysis if clinically indicated (IDSA 2013)

f. Evaluation if surgery is performed (AAOS 2010, IDSA 2013)

  i. Use frozen sections of periprosthetic tissues when reoperation performed and diagnosis of infection uncertain; presence of inflammation on histology is highly suggestive of infection

  ii. Obtain multiple cultures (3–6) during reoperation

g. Interpretation of results

  i. AAOS 2012: A definite PJI exists when:

    1. There is a draining sinus tract, or

    2. A pathogen is isolated from ≥2 samples, or

    3. ≥4 of the following exist:

      a. ESR and CRP are elevated

      b. Synovial WBC is elevated

      c. Synovial polymorphonuclear proportion (PMN %) is elevated

      d. Gross purulence is present in the joint

      e. Organism is isolated from a single sample

TABLE 6-7

DECISION TREE TO ASSESS SUSPECTED INFECTED HIP			
Suspicion of Infection	**ESR or CRP Elevated**	**Planned Reoperation**	**Recommended Test**
High	One or both	Planned or not	Aspiration
Low	One or both	Planned	Aspiration or frozen section
Low	Both	Not planned	Aspiration
Low	One	Not planned	Reevaluate in ≤3 months
Either	Neither	Planned or not	None

Source: Adapted from AAOS 2010.

        f. 5 PMNs in each of 5 high power fields (400 × magnification) on histology

   ii. IDSA 2013: A definite PJI exists when:

      1. There is a draining sinus tract

      2. There is purulence surrounding the prosthesis without other known etiology

      3. Definitive evidence of PJI if ≥2 cultures for operation or aspiration yield the same organism (genus/species/antibiogram), or a single culture is positive for a virulent organism (e.g., *S. aureus*)

  iii. A PJI may still be present even if above criteria are not met (AAOS 2012, IDSA 2013)

  iv. Isolation of single organism which is also a common contaminant (e.g., *Propionibacterium acnes*) may not be evidence of infection, but also may cause low-grade infection which may not routinely cause abnormal labs (AAOS 2012, IDSA 2013)

Acute Medical Management

1. Antimicrobial therapy (AAOS 2010)

  a. Withhold antibiotic treatment until after cultures are obtained

  b. Give prophylactic preoperative antibiotics to patients with PJI who are undergoing reoperation

2. Choice of antibiotic (IDSA 2013)

  a. Following debridement and retention of prosthesis:

    i. *Staphylococcus* infection: 2–6 weeks of pathogen specific IV agent with rifampin 300–450 mg PO BID, followed by rifampin + oral agent; see Table 6-8 for recommended agents

      1. Total therapy 3 months for THA, total elbow/shoulder/ankle infections

      2. Total therapy 6 months for total knee arthroplasty (TKA)

      3. If rifampin cannot be used, give 4–6 weeks of pathogen-specific IV agents

    ii. Infection with other organisms: 4–6 weeks of pathogen-specific IV or oral antimicrobial therapy (Table 6-8)

  b. Following 1-stage exchange

    i. *Staphylococcus* infection: 2–6 weeks of pathogen specific IV agent with rifampin 300–450 mg PO BID, followed by rifampin + oral agent for 3 months total therapy (Table 6-8)

    ii. Infection with other organisms: 4–6 weeks of pathogen-specific IV or oral agent (Table 6-8)

  c. Following resection (with or without planned 2-stage): 4–6 weeks of pathogen-specific IV or PO agent (Table 6-8)

TABLE 6-8

PATHOGEN-SPECIFIC ANTIMICROBIALS FOR PROSTHETIC JOINT INFECTION

Pathogen	Preferred	Alternatives	Notes
Staphylococcus (oxacillin susceptible)	Nafcillin 1.5–2 g IV q4–6 h Cefazolin 1–2 g IV q8 h Ceftriaxone 1–2 g IV q24 h Oral agent with and following IV: Rifampin 300–450 mg PO BID Oral agent with rifampin, following IV: Ciprofloxacin Levofloxacin	Vancomycin 15 mg/kg IV q12 h Daptomycin 6 mg/kg IV q24 h Linezolid 600 mg PO/IV q12 h Trimethoprim/sulfamethoxazole Minocycline/doxycycline Cephalexin Dicloxacillin	Duration 2–6 weeks with rifampin, then oral agent with rifampin × 3–6 months If unable to use rifampin, use parenteral antimicrobial only for 4–6 weeks
Staphylococcus (oxacillin resistant)	Vancomycin 15 mg/kg IV q12 h	Daptomycin 6 mg/kg IV q24 h Linezolid 600 mg PO/IV q12 h	See text in Acute Medical Management for companion use of rifampin and subsequent oral agents for susceptible PJI
Enterococcus spp. (penicillin susceptible)	Penicillin G 20–24 million units IV q24 h continuous or ÷ 6 Ampicillin 12 g IV q24 h continuous or ÷ 6	Vancomycin 15 mg/kg IV q12 h Daptomycin 6 mg/kg IV q24 h Linezolid 600 mg PO/IV q12 h	Vancomycin for penicillin allergic only Consider addition of aminoglycoside
Enterococcus spp. (penicillin resistant)	Vancomycin 15 mg/kg IV q12 h	Daptomycin 6 mg/kg IV q24 h Linezolid 600 mg PO/IV q12 h	Consider addition of aminoglycoside
Pseudomonas aeruginosa	Cefepime 2 g IV q12 h Meropenem 1 g IV q8 h	Ciprofloxacin 750 mg PO BID or 400 mg IV q12 h Ceftazidime 2 g IV q8 h	Consider addition of aminoglycoside Consider 2 drug coverage (one drug may be in spacer)

(Continued)

TABLE 6-8 (Continued)

PATHOGEN-SPECIFIC ANTIMICROBIALS FOR PROSTHETIC JOINT INFECTION			
Pathogen	**Preferred**	**Alternatives**	**Notes**
Enterobacter spp.	Cefepime 2 g IV q12 h Ertapenem 1 g IV q24 h	Ciprofloxacin 750 mg PO BID or 400 mg IV q12 h	
Enterobacteriaceae	IV β-lactam per sensitivities Ciprofloxacin 750 mg PO BID		
β-hemolytic *Streptococcus*	Penicillin G 20–24 million units IV q24 h continuous or ÷ 6 Ceftriaxone 2 g IV q24 h	Vancomycin 15 mg/kg IV q12 h	Vancomycin for penicillin allergic only
Propionibacterium acnes	Penicillin G 20 million units IV q24 h continuous or ÷ 6 Ceftriaxone 2 g IV q24 h	Clindamycin 600–900 mg IV q8 h Or 300–450 mg PO QID Vancomycin 15 mg/kg IV q12 h	

[1]Follow guidelines for antibiotic dosing adjustments based on patient renal and hepatic function, serum levels, in vitro sensitivities, patient allergies, potential drug interactions, contraindications; e.g., risk of QTc prolongation and tendon rupture with fluoroquinolones.
Source: IDSA 2013; Table 2.

    d. Following amputation

        i. 24–48 hours following surgery; if sepsis or bacteremia were present, treat appropriately

        ii. 4–6 weeks IV or PO if residual infected bone or soft tissue present

3. Select oral agents that are highly bioavailable

Interventions

1. Approach to surgical decision (IDSA 2013)

    a. Orthopedic surgeon guides initial management with appropriate infectious disease, plastic surgery, and other specialty consultation as necessary

    b. Surgical strategy for patient with diagnosed PJI (IDSA 2013)

        i. Orthopedic literature provides some detailed algorithms regarding surgical strategies, which are not part of established guidelines; one such strategy is outlined in the source AAOS 2012

        ii. Duration of symptoms <3 weeks or prosthesis age <30 days

            1. If prosthesis well fixed, no sinus tract, and infection susceptible to oral antibiotics, proceed with debridement and retention of prosthesis

            2. If not all of the above, remove prosthesis

            3. If patient has total hip arthroplasty (THA), adequate soft tissue and bone stock (with no bone graft required), and known organism susceptible to appropriate oral agents, Proceed to 1-stage exchange (immediate replacement of prosthesis)

            4. If not all of c., and patient has no prior 2-stage exchange with infection or failure, delayed re-implantation is feasible, and anticipated good functional outcome, proceed with 2-stage exchange

            5. If not all of d., and there is no inadequate tissue following necrotizing fasciitis, no severe bone loss, adequate soft tissue for coverage, medical therapy is available, and there would be functional benefit, proceed to resection arthroplasty or arthrodesis

            6. If patient comorbidities or preference contraindicates surgery, proceed to medical therapy only

            7. Otherwise, consider amputation or referral to a specialty hospital

Management After Stabilization (IDSA 2013)

1. Use tissue cultures and cultures from ultrasonication of resected prostheses to guide antimicrobial therapy following resection arthroplasty

2. Consider chronic suppression with oral antibiotics after treatment above, mainly for patients who refuse or are not candidates for further reimplantation, revision, excision arthroplasty, or amputation

3. See Table 6-9 for antimicrobials used for chronic suppression, if indicated

Sources:

1. IDSA 2013: Osmon DR, Berbari EF, Berendt AR, et al. Diagnosis and management of prosthetic joint infection: clinical practice guidelines by the Infectious Diseases Society of America. Clin Infect Dis. 2013;56(1):1–10. [https://www.ncbi.nlm.nih.gov/pubmed/23223583]
2. AAOS 2010: American Academy of Orthopaedic Surgeons; The diagnosis of periprosthetic joint infections of the hip and knee. Guideline and evidence report. AAOS clinical practice guidelines unit. 2010 June. [https://www.aaos.org/Research/guidelines/PJIguideline.pdf]

TABLE 6-9

ORAL ANTIMICROBIALS USED FOR CHRONIC SUPPRESSION OF PJI[1]		
Pathogen	Preferred	Alternatives
Staphylococcus (oxacillin susceptible)	Cephalexin 500 mg PO TID or QID Cefadroxil 500 mg PO BID	Dicloxacillin 500 mg PO TID or QID Clindamycin 300 mg PO QID Amoxicillin-clavulanate 500 mg PO TID
Staphylococcus (oxacillin resistant)	Trimethoprim-sulfamethoxazole DS 1 tab PO BID Minocycline/doxycycline 100 mg PO BID	
β-hemolytic *Streptococcus*	Penicillin V 500 mg PO BID-QID Amoxicillin 500 mg PO TID	Cephalexin 500 mg PO TID or QID
Enterococcus spp. (penicillin susceptible)	Penicillin V 500 mg PO BID-QID Amoxicillin 500 mg PO TID	
Pseudomonas aeruginosa	Ciprofloxacin 250–500 mg PO BID	
Enterobacteriaceae	Trimethoprim-sulfamethoxazole DS 1 tab PO BID	β-lactam per sensitivities
Propionibacterium acnes	Penicillin V 500 mg PO BID-QID Amoxicillin 500 mg PO TID	Cephalexin 500 mg PO TID or QID Minocycline/doxycycline 100 mg PO BID

[1]Follow guidelines for antibiotic dosing adjustments based on patient renal and hepatic function, serum levels, in vitro sensitivities, patient allergies, potential drug interactions, contraindications, e.g., risk of QTc prolongation and tendon rupture with fluoroquinolones.

Abbreviations: g, grams; IV, intravenous; PO, orally; ÷ 6, in 6 divided doses; q8 h, every 8 hours; BID, 2 times daily; TID, 3 times daily; QID, 4 times daily.

Source: IDSA 2013; Table 3.

CANDIDIASIS

Initial Assessment (IDSA 2016)

1. Diagnosis
   a. Cultures are not sufficiently sensitive[14]; blood cultures may take days to weeks to turn positive
   b. Consider antigen and antibody testing[15]
   c. Consider β-D-glucan[16] assay as an adjunct to cultures
      i. Positive results suggest the possibility of invasive fungal infection but are not specific for invasive candidiasis
      ii. May identify invasive candidiasis weeks to days before positive blood cultures
      iii. Sensitivity of 75%–80% and specificity of 80%
      iv. False positives may be caused by bacteremia, certain antibiotics, hemodialysis, fungal colonization, albumin or IVIG treatment, use of surgical gauze containing β-D-glucan, and mucositis
   d. Consider *Candida* PCR assays as adjunct to cultures
      i. Pooled sensitivity and specificity in suspected invasive candidiasis is 95% and 92%, respectively
      ii. Limitations include lack of standardized methodologies and multicenter validation of assay performance

Acute Medical Management

1. Candidemia, nonneutropenic patients
   a. Give initial therapy with an echinocandin (caspofungin 70 mg loading dose then 50 mg daily, micafungin 100 mg daily, anidulafungin 200 mg loading dose then 100 mg daily)
      i. Alternative[17]: Fluconazole (IV/PO) 800 mg (12 mg/kg) loading dose then 400 mg (6 mg/kg) daily
      ii. Alternative: Voriconazole 400 (6 mg/kg) twice daily × 2 doses then 200 mg (3 mg/kg) twice daily; effective but no better than fluconazole
      iii. Test for echinocandin susceptibility in patients who have had prior echinocandin therapy before or those infected with *C. glabrata* or *C. pampilosis*
      iv. Test for azole susceptibility in all bloodstream and other clinically relevant *Candida* isolates

---

[14]Sensitivity of blood cultures: 50%. Sensitivity of tissue or fluid cultures: <50%.
[15]Serum IgG responses against specific antigens have performed better than IgM. *Candida* antigens are cleared rapidly from the bloodstream. This practice is more prevalent in Europe than the United States.
[16]A cell wall component of *Candida* species, *Aspergillus* species, *Pneumocystis jiroveci*, and several other fungi.
[17]Acceptable in those who are not critically ill and are considered unlikely to have fluconazole-resistant *Candida*.

    b. Transition from echinocandin to azole within 5–7 days if patients are clinically stable, have azole susceptible *Candida* species, and negative repeat blood cultures after initiation of antifungal therapy

    c. *C. glabrata*

        i. Transition to higher dose fluconazole 800 mg (12 mg/kg) daily or voriconazole 200–300 mg (3–4 mg/kg) twice daily (if azole susceptible)

        ii. Consider lipid formulation amphotericin B (3–5 mg/kg daily) as alternative if there is intolerance, limited availability, or resistance to other antifungal agents

        iii. Transition to fluconazole within 5–7 days if acceptable to do so

        iv. Transition to voriconazole for step-down oral therapy for *C. krusei*

    d. Suspected azole- and echinocandin-resistant *Candida* infections: Give lipid formulation amphotericin B (3–5 mg/kg daily)

    e. Obtain dilated ophthalmological exam by an ophthalmologist within a week of diagnosis

    f. Get follow-up blood cultures daily or every 48 hours to establish clearance of the candidemia

    g. Duration of therapy: 2 weeks after documented clearance of *Candida*, assuming resolution of symptoms attributed to candidemia and no obvious metastatic complications

    h. Remove CVCs as soon as possible when the source is presumed to be the CVC

2. Candidemia, neutropenic patients

    a. Give initial therapy with echinocandin[18]

        i. Alternative: Lipid formulation amphotericin B[18] is effective but has more potential for toxicity

        ii. Alternative: Fluconazole,[18] in those who are not critically ill and have had no prior exposure to azoles

    b. Step-down therapy in clinically stable patients with persistent neutropenia with susceptible isolates and documented bloodstream clearance

        i. Fluconazole 400 mg (6 mg/kg) daily AND

        ii. Voriconazole 400 mg (6 mg/kg) twice daily × 2 doses, then 200–300 mg (3–4 mg/kg) twice daily

    c. Consider voriconazole for additional mold coverage when needed

    d. *C. krusei*: Use echinocandin, lipid formulation amphotericin B, or voriconazole

    e. Duration of therapy: At least 2 weeks after documented clearance of *Candida* from the bloodstream, assuming resolution of neutropenia/symptoms from candidemia and no metastatic complications

---

[18]Same doses as nonneutropenic patients.

    f. Obtain dilated funduscopic examination in the first week after recovery from neutropenia[19]

    g. CVC: Less likely to be the source in neutropenia; consider catheter removal on an individual basis

    h. Consider GCSF-mobilized granulocyte transfusion in persistent candidemia with anticipated prolonged neutropenia

3. Chronic disseminated (hepatosplenic) candidiasis

    a. Initial therapy

        i. Lipid formulation amphotericin B or echinocandin for several weeks

        ii. Transition to oral fluconazole 400 mg (6 mg/kg) daily in patients who are unlikely to have fluconazole-resistant isolate

        iii. Duration of therapy: Until lesions resolve on imaging, usually several months

        iv. Do not delay chemotherapy or hematopoietic cell transplantation due to chronic disseminated candidiasis; continue antifungal therapy throughout the period of high risk to prevent relapse

        v. Consider 1–2-week course of NSAIDs or corticosteroids in those with debilitating persistent fevers

4. Nonneutropenic patients with suspected invasive candidiasis in the ICU

    a. Preferred empiric therapy: Echinocandin

        i. Alternative: Fluconazole if no recent azole exposure and not colonized with azole-resistant *Candida*

        ii. Alternative: Lipid formulation amphotericin B if there is intolerance to other antifungal agents

        iii. Duration of therapy: 2 weeks if there is improvement

    b. If there is no clinical response to empiric antifungal therapy at 4–5 days and no subsequent evidence of invasive candidiasis or there is a negative nonculture based diagnostic assay with high NPV, consider stopping antifungal therapy

5. Intra-abdominal candidiasis

    a. Risk factors: Recent abdominal surgery, anastomotic leaks, necrotizing pancreatitis

    b. Treatment includes source control and appropriate drainage/ debridement

    c. Treat the same as for the nonneutropenic patient

    d. Duration of therapy: Determined by adequacy of source control and clinical response

6. *Candida* in the respiratory tract is usually colonization and rarely requires antifungal treatment

---

[19]Ophthalmological findings of choroidal and vitreal infection are minimal and difficult to diagnose until neutropenia resolves.

7. Intravascular candidiasis
    a. Native valve endocarditis
        i. Antifungals: Lipid formulation amphotericin B with or without flucytosine 25 mg/kg 4× daily or high-dose echinocandin (caspofungin 150 mg daily, micafungin 150 mg daily, or anidulafungin 200 mg daily)
        ii. Step-down therapy to fluconazole if susceptible, clinically stable, and bloodstream cleared; use voriconazole or posaconazole (300 mg daily) if not susceptible to fluconazole
        iii. Pursue valve replacement; continue treatment for at least 6 weeks after surgery or longer if there are other complications including perivalvular abscess formation
        iv. If unable to undergo valve replacement, give long-term suppression with fluconazole 400–800 mg daily
    b. Prosthetic valve endocarditis: Same antifungal regimen as native valve endocarditis; chronic suppression with fluconazole to prevent recurrence
    c. Pacemaker/ICD infection: Remove the entire device; antifungal therapy as for native valve endocarditis
        i. Infections limited to generator pockets: Duration 4 weeks after device removal
        ii. Infections including the wires: Duration at least 6 weeks after wire removal
        iii. VAD that cannot be removed: Chronic suppressive therapy with fluconazole while the device remains in place
8. Suppurative thrombophlebitis
    a. Catheter removal, I&D, or resection of vein
    b. Lipid formulation amphotericin B, fluconazole, or echinocandin for at least 2 weeks after candidemia has cleared
    c. Step down to fluconazole if able
    d. If clinically stable, discontinue therapy once thrombus has resolved
9. *Candida* endophthalmitis
    a. Ophthalmologist to determine the extent of the infection (anterior/posterior eye segments, macula, vitreous involvement)
    b. *Candida* chorioretinitis without vitritis: Fluconazole or voriconazole
        i. Liposomal amphotericin B with or without oral flucytosine if resistant to fluconazole/voriconazole
        ii. Macular involvement: Add intravitreal injection of amphotericin B deoxycholate, 5–10 μg/0.1 mL sterile water, or voriconazole 100 μg/0.1 mL sterile water or NS to ensure a prompt high level of antifungal activity
        iii. Duration of therapy: At least 4–6 weeks and until repeat ophthalmological exam shows resolution of lesions

    c. *Candida* chorioretinitis with vitritis: Same as without vitritis with macular involvement: Consider vitrectomy; same duration of therapy

10. Central nervous system candidiasis

    a. Initial treatment: Liposomal amphotericin B 5 mg/kg daily with or without oral flucytosine 25 mg/kg 4×/day

    b. Step-down therapy after initial response to treatment: Fluconazole

    c. Duration of therapy: Until all signs and symptoms and CSF/radiological abnormalities have resolved

    d. Remove infected CNS devices if possible; if a ventricular device cannot be removed, give amphotericin B deoxycholate through the device into the ventricle (0.01–0.5 mg in 2 mL 5% dextrose in water)

11. *Candida* urinary tract infections

    a. Eliminate predisposing factors (e.g., indwelling catheters) if possible

    b. Do not treat unless the patient is at high risk[20]

        i. Neutropenia treatment is the same as candidemia

        ii. If undergoing urologic manipulation, give oral fluconazole 400 mg daily or amphotericin B deoxycholate 0.3–0.6 mg/kg daily, several days before and after the procedure

    c. Symptomatic *Candida* cystitis: Fluconazole 200 mg (3 mg/kg) daily × 2 weeks

        i. If fluconazole-resistant *C. glabrata*: Amphotericin B deoxycholate 0.3–0.6 mg/kg daily for 1–7 days or oral flucytosine 25 mg/kg 4×/day for 7–10 days

        ii. *C. krusei*: Amphotericin B deoxycholate 0.3–0.6 mg/kg daily for 1–7 days

        iii. Remove indwelling bladder catheter if able; amphotericin B deoxycholate bladder irrigation (50 mg/L sterile water daily × 5 days) may be helpful

    d. Symptomatic ascending *Candida* pyelonephritis: Fluconazole 200–400 mg daily × 2 weeks

        i. Fluconazole-resistant *C. glabrata*: Amphotericin B deoxycholate 0.3–0.6 mg/kg daily for 1–7 days with or without oral flucytosine 25 mg/kg 4×x/day

        ii. *C. krusei*: Amphotericin B deoxycholate 0.3–0.6 mg/kg daily for 1–7 days

        iii. Eliminate urinary tract obstruction; consider removal or replacement of nephrostomy tubes or stents if in place

    e. *Candida* UTI associated with fungus balls: Surgical intervention with the same antifungal regimen as above

---

[20] Neutropenia, patients who will undergo urologic manipulation.

       i. Irrigate through nephrostomy tubes (if present) with amphotericin B deoxycholate 25–50 mg in 200–500 mL sterile water

12. Vulvovaginal candidiasis
    a. Uncomplicated: Topical antifungal agent, no one agent is superior
        i. Alternative: Oral fluconazole 150 mg once
    b. Severe: Fluconazole 150 mg every 72 hours for 2–3 doses
    c. *C. glabrata* unresponsive to azoles: Topical intravaginal boric acid in gelatin capsules, 600 mg daily × 14 days
        i. Alternative: Nystatin intravaginal suppository 100,000 U daily × 14 days
        ii. Topical 17% flucytosine cream with or without 3% amphotericin B cream daily × 14 days
    d. Recurrent: 10–14 days of induction therapy with topical agent or oral fluconazole, followed by fluconazole 150 mg weekly × 6 months

13. Oropharyngeal candidiasis
    a. Mild: Clotrimazole troches 10 mg 5×/day or miconazole mucoadhesive buccal 50 mg tab to the mucosal surface over the canine fossa daily ×7–14 days
        i. Alternative: Nystatin (100,000 U/mL) 4–6 mL 4×/day or 1–2 nystatin pastilles (200,000 U each) 4×/day for 7–14 days
    b. Moderate to severe: Oral fluconazole 100–200 mg daily × 7–14 days
    c. Fluconazole-resistant disease: Itraconazole solution 200 mg daily or posaconazole suspension 400 mg twice daily × 3 days, then 400 mg daily for up to 28 days
        i. Alternative: Voriconazole 200 mg twice daily or amphotericin B deoxycholate oral suspension 100 mg/mL 4×/day
        ii. IV echinocandin or IV amphotericin deoxycholate also alternatives for refractory disease
    d. Chronic suppressive therapy is usually not necessary, but if needed, give fluconazole 100 mg 3×/week
    e. HIV-infected patients: Give ART to reduce recurrent infections
    f. Denture-related candidiasis: Disinfection of the dentures and antifungal therapy

14. Esophageal candidiasis
    a. Systemic antifungal therapy always required; trial of diagnostic antifungal therapy is appropriate prior to endoscopic exam
    b. Fluconazole 200–400 mg daily × 14–21 days
        i. If oral therapy not tolerated, use IV fluconazole 400 mg daily or echinocandin (micafungin 150 mg daily, caspofungin 70 mg loading dose then 50 mg daily, or anidulafungin 200 mg daily)
        ii. Less preferred alternative: Amphotericin B deoxycholate 0.3–0.7 mg/kg daily

  iii. De-escalate to oral fluconazole when able to tolerate oral intake

 c. Fluconazole-refractory disease: Itraconazole solution 200 mg daily or voriconazole 200 mg twice daily (IV/PO) × 14–21 days

  i. Alternatives: Echinocandin × 7–14 days or amphotericin B deoxycholate × 21 days; posaconazole suspension 400 mg twice daily or ER tabs 300 mg daily can be considered as well

 d. Recurrent esophagitis: Consider chronic suppressive therapy with fluconazole 100–200 mg 3×/week

 e. HIV-infected patients: Give ART to reduce recurrent infections

15. Prophylaxis against invasive candidiasis in the ICU

 a. Use fluconazole 800 mg (12 mg/kg) loading dose then 400 mg (6 mg/kg) daily in high-risk patients in adult ICUs that have a >5% rate of invasive candidiasis

 b. Alternative: Echinocandin

 c. Daily chlorhexidine baths decrease incidence of bloodstream infections, including candidemia

Source:

1. Clinical practice guidelines for the management of candidiasis: 2016 update by the IDSA. CID (December 2015).

OUTPATIENT PARENTERAL ANTIBIOTIC THERAPY

Initial Assessment

1. Outpatient parenteral antibiotic therapy (OPAT) is effective for a wide variety of infections

 a. OPAT: Provision of parenteral antimicrobial therapy in at least two doses on different days without intervening hospitalization

 b. Outpatient: Home, physician offices, hospital-based ambulatory care, ED, hemodialysis units, infusion centers, SNF, long-term care facilities, rehabilitation centers

 c. Parenteral: Intravenous, subcutaneous, intramuscular

2. Assess patient's general medical condition, the infectious process, and the home situation before initiating OPAT

 a. Is the parenteral antimicrobial needed?

 b. Do the patient's medical care needs exceed available resources at the proposed site of care?

 c. Is the home/outpatient environment safe and adequate to support care?[21]

---

[21]Specifically evaluate IV drug use and alcohol abuse before initiating OPAT. Patients likely to abuse vascular access are poor candidates for OPAT.

   d. Are the patient/caregivers willing to participate and able to safely, effectively, and reliably delivery IV antimicrobial therapy?

   e. Are methods for rapid and reliable communication about problems/monitoring of therapy in place between members of the OPAT team?

   f. Does the patient/caregiver understand the risk/benefits/economic considerations involved in OPAT?

   g. Does informed consent need to be documented?

3. Assemble OPAT team including physician,[22] nursing, pharmacy, allied health care professionals,[23] and case manager/billing staff

   a. Physician responsibilities include establishing a diagnosis, prescribing treatment, determining appropriate site of care, monitoring during therapy, and assuring overall quality of care

Management After Stabilization

1. Antimicrobial selection for OPAT is different from inpatient antimicrobial therapy

   a. Prefer once-daily regimens

2. Consider potential adverse effects and antimicrobial stability (see Table 6-10)

3. Give the first dose in a supervised setting; monitor labs and clinical status regularly while on OPAT (see Table 6-11)

Source:

1. IDSA 2004: Tice AD, Rehm SJ, Dalovisio JR, et al. Practice guidelines for outpatient parenteral antimicrobial therapy. Clin Infect Dis. 2004;38:1651–1672. [http://www.idsociety.org/uploadedFiles/IDSA/Guidelines-Patient_Care/PDF_Library/OPAT.pdf]

NEW FEVER IN THE CRITICALLY ILL ADULT

Initial Assessment

1. Defining fever

   a. Many definitions of fever

      i. Core temp >38.0°C

      ii. Two consecutive temperatures >38.3°C

      iii. Temperature >38.0°C for >1 hour

      iv. Single oral temperature >38.3°C (in neutropenia)

---

[22]Infectious disease specialist or physician knowledgeable about infectious diseases and the use of antimicrobials in OPAT, as well as primary care physicians.

[23]Physical therapist, dietician, occupational therapist, social worker.

TABLE 6-10

PROPERTIES OF COMMONLY PRESCRIBED ANTIMICROBIALS

Drug	Half-Life (h)	Optimal Dilution (mg/mL)	Stability at −20°C	Stability at 5°C	Stability at 25°C	Phlebitis Risk[1]/ Other
Acyclovir	2–3.5	5	–	37 days	>37 days	1/Do not refrigerate
Amphotericin B	24–360	0.1	–	35 days	5 days	3
Liposomal amphotericin B	24–360	4		24 hours	5 days	2
Amphotericin B lipid complex	24–360	1	–	48 hours	6 hours	2
Ampicillin	1	30		48 hours	8 hours	2
Ampicillin-sulbactam	1	20	–	48 hours	8 hours	2
Caspofungin	>48	0.2–0.3	–	24 hours	1 day	1
Cefazolin	1–2	10–20	30 days	10 days	1 day	1
Cefoperazone	1.5–25	40	96 days	80 days	80 days	1
Ceftazidime	1.4–2	1–40	90 days	21 days	2 days	1
Ceftriaxone	5.4–10.9	10–40	180 days	10 days	3 days	1
Cefuroxime	1–2	5–10	30 days	180 days	1 day	1
Chloramphenicol	1.5–4	10–20	180 days	30 days	30 days	1
Clindamycin	2–3	6–12	56 days	48 hours	3 days	1
Doxycycline	22–24	0.1–1	56 days	48 hours	3 days	2/Protect from sunlight

(Continued)

TABLE 6-10 (Continued)

PROPERTIES OF COMMONLY PRESCRIBED ANTIMICROBIALS

Drug	Half-Life (h)	Optimal Dilution (mg/mL)	Stability at −20°C	Stability at 5°C	Stability at 25°C	Phlebitis Risk[1]/Other
Erythromycin	1.5–2	0.1–0.2	30 days	14 days	1 day	3
Ertapenem	4	20	–	24 hours	6 hours	2
Ganciclovir	2.5–3.6	5	364 days	35 days	5 days	1
Gentamicin	2–3	0.6–1	30 days	30 days	30 days	1
Imipenem-cilastatin	0.8–1.3	2.5–5	–	2 days	10 hours	2
Linezolid	4.5	2	–	–	–	1
Meropenem	1.5	5–20	-	24 hours	4 hours	1
Nafcillin	0.5–1.5	2–40	90 days	3 days	1 day	3
Oxacillin	0.3–0.8	10–100	30 days	7 days	1 day	2
Penicillin G	0.4–0.9	0.2	84 days	14 days	2 days	2/Degradation products can form in a few hours
Quinupristin-dalfopristin	3/1	2	-	54 hours	5 hours	3
TMP-SMX	8–11/10–13	8	-	–	6 hours	2
Tobramycin	2–3	0.2–3.2	30 days	4 days	2 days	1
Vancomycin	4–6	5	63 days	63 days	7 days	2

[1]Degree of tendency to cause phlebitis: 1: mild; 2: moderate; 3: high. Affects the type of VAD used for OPAT.

Source: IDSA 2004, Table 5.

TABLE 6-11

TYPES OF VASCULAR ACCESS DEVICES FOR OPAT

Device	Characteristics
Peripheral short catheter	Short course (<2 weeks for adults, <1 week for children) of agents with low risk for phlebitis in patients with good vein status
Midline catheter	Course >1 week, patients with moderately difficult venous access
PICC	Prolonged course >1–2 weeks, risks of other types of central lines no warranted; compatible with programmable pumps
Central catheter (tunneled/nontunneled)	Longer term access, infusion of irritative agents; may be preferred over PICC in active patients/infants/children needing frequent blood draws; implantable ports not commonly used

Source: Adapted from IDSA 2004.

    b. Most accurate methods for temperature measurement: Pulmonary artery thermistor, urinary bladder catheter thermistor, esophageal probe, and rectal probe

        i. Other acceptable methods: Oral probe, infrared ear thermometry

        ii. Less desirable methods: Temporal artery thermometer, axillary thermometer, chemical dot

    c. Patients with an infection are not always febrile[24]

    d. Other potential signs and symptoms of infection include hypotension, tachycardia, tachypnea, altered mental status, rigors, skin lesions, respiratory distress, oliguria, lactic acidosis, leukocytosis, leukopenia, bandemia, thrombocytopenia, etc.

  2. Blood cultures

    a. Draw 3–4 blood cultures within the first 24 hours of the onset of fever, ideally before initiation of antimicrobial therapy

        i. Draw additional blood cultures (in pairs) thereafter when there is clinical suspicion for continuing for recurrent bacteremia/fungemia or for test of cure, 48–96 hours after initiation of appropriate antimicrobial therapy

        ii. Use proper skin antiseptic (2% chlorhexidine gluconate in 70% isopropyl alcohol, >30 seconds of drying time)

        iii. If the patient has an intravascular catheter, draw at least one blood culture through the catheter and at least one by venipuncture

---

[24]The elderly, patients with open abdominal wounds, large burns, on ECMO or CRRT, patients with CHF, ESLD, or ESRD, patients on anti-inflammatory or antipyretic medications may not be able to mount fevers.

3. Management of intravascular catheters
   a. Examine catheter sites for evidence of infection, venous thrombosis, or embolic phenomena at least once daily
      i. Gram stain and culture any purulence at the insertion site
      ii. Remove any catheters with suspicion for infection, embolic phenomena, or vascular compromise; replace at a different site
   b. If a catheter-related infection is suspected, remove the catheter and send for culture; obtain blood cultures[25]; do not routinely culture all catheters removed from ICU patients
4. Evaluation of the pulmonary tract
   a. Obtain chest imaging: Upright AP CXR in most cases, but obtain 2-view PA/lateral CXR or CT scan to obtain more information, especially in immunocompromised patients
   b. Obtain a lower respiratory tract secretion sample[26] before initiation or change in antimicrobials
      i. Process samples within 2 hours
      ii. Obtain Gram stain and culture for all samples; consider additional testing, guided by clinical status and epidemiological factors
   c. Obtain pleural fluid with ultrasound guidance for Gram stain and culture if there is an adjacent infiltrate or another reason to suspect infection and the fluid can be safely aspirated
5. Evaluation of the gastrointestinal tract
   a. If >2 stools/day that conform to the container in a patient with risk factors for C. difficile who has clinical indication for further evaluation:
      i. Send one stool sample for C. difficile common antigen, EIA for toxin A and B, or tissue culture assay
         1. If the EIA is negative, send a second sample for EIA testing
         2. Second sample not necessary if the common antigen test was negative
      ii. If severe illness is present and no rapid tests are available, consider flexible sigmoidoscopy for diagnosis
      iii. If severe illness is present, consider empirical oral vancomycin therapy while awaiting diagnosis
      iv. Stool cultures for other enteric pathogens are rarely indicated in patients who did not present to the hospital with diarrhea or are HIV negative; send stool cultures if epidemiologically indicated or patient is immunocompromised
      v. Consider stool for norovirus if clinically indicated

---

[25] At least two blood cultures: One from the suspected catheter and the other from a peripheral venipuncture.
[26] Expectorated sputum, induced sputum, tracheal secretions, bronchoscopic or nonbronchoscopic alveolar lavage.

6. Evaluation of the urinary tract
   a. If high risk for UTI[27] and symptoms of a UTI, send urine for microscopy, Gram stain, and culture
      i. Patients with urinary catheters should have urine collected from the sampling port of the catheter (not the drainage bag)
      ii. Sample should be processed within 1 hour; otherwise, it should be refrigerated
      iii. Dipstick tests are not recommended for use in patients with urinary catheters
   b. Catheter specimen cultures with $>10^3$ cfu/mL represent true bacteriuria/candiduria, but lower concentrations do not commonly cause fever

7. Evaluation of the facial sinuses
   a. If clinically indicated, obtain CT scan of the facial sinuses
   b. If the patient does not respond to empiric therapy, puncture and aspirate the involved sinuses under antiseptic conditions; send aspirated fluid for Gram stain and culture for aerobic/anaerobic bacteria and fungi for ID and sensitivities

8. Evaluation of fever within 72 hours of surgery
   a. CXR and urinalysis/culture are not mandatory if the only indication is fever; send urinalysis/culture if the patient has had an indwelling bladder catheter >72 hours
   b. Examine surgical wounds daily for evidence of infection; culture only if there are signs and symptoms suggestive for infection
   c. Maintain a high level of suspicion for VTE[28]

9. Evaluation for surgical site infection
   a. Examine surgical incision daily for erythema, purulence, or tenderness
      i. If there is suspicion for infection, open and culture the incision
         1. Prefer tissue biopsies/aspirates over swabs
         2. Drainage from superficial surgical site infections may not require Gram stain/culture because incision, drainage, and antibiotic therapy may not be required
         3. Avoid superficial swab cultures; they are likely to be contaminated with skin flora

10. Evaluation of the central nervous system
    a. If altered mentation or focal neurologic signs are unexplained, consider lumbar puncture with a new fever, unless otherwise contraindicated; if focal neurologic findings suggest disease above the foramen magnum, proceed with an imaging study before the lumbar puncture; if a mass is present, obtain neurology/neurosurgery consultation

---

[27] Kidney transplant patients, granulocytopenic patients, patients with recent urologic surgery or obstruction.

[28] Especially in patients who are sedentary, have lower limb immobility, have malignancy, or are on oral contraceptives.

    b. In patients with an intracranial device, collect CSF from the CSF reservoir; if CSF flow to the subarachnoid space, also obtain CSF from the lumbar space; in patients with ventriculostomies who develop stupor or signs of meningitis, remove the catheter and culture the tip

    c. Evaluate CSF by Gram stain, culture, glucose, protein, and cell count with differential; consider additional testing dictated by clinical situation

11. Other considerations

    a. Post-transfusion infections with EBV or CMV

    b. "Silent sources of infection": Otitis media, decubitus ulcers, retained foreign bodies, infected hardware/drains/devices

    c. Serum procalcitonin levels and endotoxin activity assay can be used as an adjunctive diagnostic tool for discriminating infection as the cause for fever or sepsis (see Table 3-3)

12. Noninfectious causes of fever in the ICU

    a. Drug fever

        i. Most notably antimicrobials (especially β-lactam drugs), antiepileptic drugs (especially phenytoin), antiarrhythmics (especially quinidine, procainamide), and antihypertensives (especially methyldopa)

        ii. Fevers induced by drugs may take several days to resolve

        iii. Withdrawal from drugs may also cause fever[29]

    b. Consider malignant hyperthermia[30] and neuroleptic malignant syndrome[31] if the fever is especially high

    c. Other causes include acalculous cholecystitis, acute myocardial infarction, adrenal insufficiency, blood transfusion reaction, cytokine-related fever, Dressler syndrome, fat emboli, ARDS, gout, heterotopic ossification, immune reconstitution inflammatory syndrome, intracranial bleed, Jarisch-Herxheimer reaction, pancreatitis, pulmonary infarction, pneumonitis without infection, stroke, thyroid storm, transplant rejection, tumor lysis syndrome, VTE

Acute Medical Management

1. Empiric therapy for new fever in the ICU

    a. If infection is clinically suggested, consider empiric antimicrobial therapy as soon as possible following collection of cultures, especially if the patient is seriously ill or deteriorating

    b. Select empiric antimicrobial therapy considering the likely pathogen source, the patient's risk for multidrug resistant pathogens, and local antimicrobial susceptibility pattern data

---

[29]Typically withdrawal from alcohol, opiates, barbiturates, and benzodiazepines.
[30]Believed to be a genetically determined response caused by succinylcholine and the inhalation anesthetics.
[31]Strongly associated with antipsychotic neuroleptic medications.

Source:

1. O'Grady NP, Barie PS, Bartlett JG, et al. Guidelines for evaluation of new fever in critically ill adult patients: 2008 update from the American College of Critical Care Medicine and the Infectious Diseases Society of America. Crit Care Med. 2008:36(4):1330–1349. [https://www.ncbi.nlm.nih.gov/pubmed/18379262]

ANTIBIOTIC STEWARDSHIP PROGRAMS

Definition (IDSA 2016)

1. Antibiotic stewardship program (ASP): Coordinated interventions designed to improve and measure the appropriate use of antibiotic agents by promoting the selection of the optimal antibiotic drug regimen including dosing, duration of therapy, and route of administration

Benefits (IDSA 2016)

1. Improved patient outcomes reduced adverse events including CDI, improvement in rates of antibiotic susceptibilities to targeted antibiotics, and optimization of resource utilization across the continuum of care

Interventions (IDSA 2016)

1. Obtain preauthorization and/or prospective audit and feedback
2. Do not rely solely on didactic educational material for stewardship[32]
3. Develop facility-specific clinical practice guidelines and a strategy to disseminate and implement them
4. Implement interventions to improve antibiotic use and clinical outcomes that target patient with specific infectious disease syndromes
5. Design ASPs to reduce the use of antibiotics associated with a high risk of *Clostridium difficile* infection
6. Encourage prescribers to perform routine review of antibiotic regimens to improve antibiotic prescribing[33]
7. Discourage antibiotic cycling as a stewardship strategy
8. Employ pharmacokinetic monitoring and adjustment programs in hospitals for aminoglycosides and vancomycin
9. In hospitalized patients, ASPs should advocate for alternative dosing strategies (vs. standard dosing) for broad-spectrum β-lactams to decrease costs
10. ASPs should work to increase appropriate use of oral antibiotics for initial therapy and timely transition from IV to oral antibiotics
11. ASPs should consider allergy assessments and PCN skin testing in patients with a history of β-lactam allergy, when appropriate[34]

[32] Passive educational activities should be used to complement other stewardship activities.
[33] Requires a methodology that includes persuasive or enforced prompting.
[34] Allergy assessments and PCN skin testing can enhance use of first-line agents but is largely unstudied as a primary ASP intervention.

12. Implement guidelines and strategies to reduce antibiotic therapy to the shortest effective duration
13. Develop stratified antibiograms to assist in empiric therapy guideline development
14. Perform raid viral testing for respiratory pathogens to reduce the use of inappropriate antibiotics
15. Perform rapid diagnostic testing in addition to conventional culture and routine reporting on blood specimens, combined with active ASP support and interpretation
16. Measure serial procalcitonin in adult ICU patient with suspected infection in order to decrease antibiotic use
17. Incorporate nonculture-based fungal markers to optimize antifungal use in patients with hematological malignancy and are at risk for invasive fungal disease
18. Monitor antibiotic use (measured as days of therapy) to assess the impact of ASPs
19. Monitor antibiotic costs based on prescriptions or administrations to best measure the impact of ASPs on expenditures
20. Consider the goals/size of the syndrome-specific intervention when measuring the impact of interventions to improve antibiotic use and clinical outcomes in patients with specific infectious disease syndromes
21. Develop facility-specific clinical guidelines for the management of febrile neutropenia in hematology-oncology patients to reduce unnecessary antibiotic use and improve outcomes
22. Use ASP interventions to improve the appropriate prescribing of antifungal treatment in immunocompromised patients
23. Implement ASP strategies in nursing homes and skilled nursing facilities to decrease unnecessary antibiotic use
24. Implement ASP strategies in NICUs to reduce inappropriate antibiotic use and/or resistance
25. Support clinicians in decisions related to antibiotic treatment in terminally ill patients

Source:

1. IDSA 2016: Barlam TF, Cosgrove SE, Abbo LM, et al. Executive summary: implementing an antibiotic stewardship program. Clin Infect Dis. 2016:62(10):1197–1202. [https://www.ncbi.nlm.nih.gov/pubmed/27118828]

Hematology

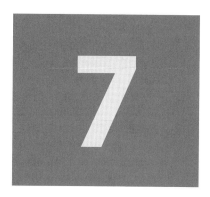

Tipu V. Khan
Seth Alkire
Samantha Chirunomula

BLOOD TRANSFUSION: INDICATIONS BY CLINICAL SETTING

Hospitalized and Critically Ill, But Hemodynamically Stable Without Coronary Artery Disease
1. AABB 2016, NICE 2014, BCSH 2012: Use restrictive rather than liberal transfusion goals[1]
2. AABB 2016
   a. Liberal Hg goal: >10 g/dL
   b. Restrictive Hg goal: >7 g/dL

Cardiac or Orthopedic Surgery Patients or Any Patient with Preexisting Cardiovascular Disease (AABB 2016)[2]
1. Transfuse to Hg >8 g/dL

Patients with Acute Coronary Syndrome
1. BCSH 2012, NICE 2014: Transfuse to Hg >8 g/dL
2. AABB 2016: Insufficient evidence to recommend liberal or restrictive strategy

Critically Ill Patients with Sepsis (BCSH 2012)
1. Transfuse to Hg >9–10 g/dL in early resuscitation
2. Transfuse to Hg >7–9 g/dL in late resuscitation

Patients with TBI and Signs of Cerebral Ischemia (BCSH 2012)
1. Transfuse to Hg >9 g/dL

Patient with Active GI Bleed (AABB 2016)
1. No recommendation made
2. Consider restrictive transfusion goal; improved 30-day mortality

---

[1]Insufficient evidence available to make blood transfusion recommendations regarding ACS, chronic thrombocytopenia, hematologic/oncologic disorders, and chronic transfusion-dependent anemia.
[2]Based on 1996 Lancet article cited in guidelines, defined as prior MI, history of angina, peripheral vascular disease, and congestive heart failure.

3. See Chapter 5, section "Upper GI Bleeding" for GI society recommendations.

Symptomatic Anemia[3] (AABB 2016)

1. Transfuse for symptomatic anemia with hemoglobin below 10 g/dL

Sources:

1. AABB 2016: Clinical practice guidelines from the AABB: red blood cell transfusion thresholds and storage, JAMA. 2016;316(19):2025–2035. [http://jamanetwork.com/journals/jama/fullarticle/2569055]
2. Effect of anemia and cardiovascular disease on surgical mortality and morbidity. Lancet. 1996;348(9034):1055–1060. [https://www.ncbi.nlm.nih.gov/pubmed/8874456]
3. BCSH 2012: Retter A, Wyncoll D, Pearse R, et al. Guidelines on the management of anaemia and red cell transfusion in adult critically ill patients. BJH. 2013;160(4):445–464. [https://www.ncbi.nlm.nih.gov/pubmed/23278459]
4. NICE 2015: National Institute for Health and Care Excellence. Blood transfusion. NICE guideline. November 18, 2015. [https://NICE.org.uk/guidance/ng24]

PLATELET TRANSFUSION: INDICATIONS BY CLINICAL SETTING

Definitions

1. 1 platelet unit = 1 apheresis unit = platelet concentrates from 4 to 6 units of pooled whole blood

Hospitalized Patients with Chemotherapy or Radiation-Induced Hypoproliferative Thrombocytopenia (AABB 2015)

1. Transfuse of 1 unit prophylactically if morning serum platelets $<10 \times 10^9$ cells/L
2. No benefit known in giving more than 1 unit, or partial units

Minor Procedures in Patients with Thrombocytopenia (AABB 2015)

1. Transfuse platelets prophylactically prior to procedure if serum platelets are below the following thresholds:
   a. Central venous catheter placement[4]: Platelets $<20 \times 10^9$ cells/L
   b. Lumbar puncture[5]: Platelets $<50 \times 10^9$ cells/L

Major Elective, Non-Neuraxial Surgery (AABB 2015)

1. Transfuse platelets prophylactically if serum platelets are $<50 \times 10^9$ cells/L

---

[3]Symptomatic anemia defined as chest pain, orthostatic hypotension, tachycardia not responsive to fluid resuscitation, and CHF.
[4]Tunneled and nontunneled CVC placements included in this recommendation.
[5]This guideline is intended for simple diagnostic/therapeutic LPs only, not intended for other procedures, including epidural anesthesia.

a. Do not routinely give prophylactic transfusions to surgical patients without thrombocytopenia unless clinical evidence of platelet dysfunction

Neuraxial Surgery (AABB 2015)

1. Customarily transfused to a pre-procedure goal of $80-100 \times 10^9$ cells/L
2. Evidence for this practice is insufficient to be included in the guidelines

Intracranial Hemorrhage (Traumatic and Spontaneous) in Patients Receiving Anti-Platelet Therapy (AABB 2015)

1. Insufficient evidence to recommend for or against routine transfusion

Acute Upper GI Bleeding

1. See Chapter 5, section "Upper GI Bleeding" for GI society recommendations.

Source:

1. Kaufman RM, Djulbegovic B, Gernsheimer T, et al. Platelet transfusion: a clinical practice guideline from the AABB. Ann Intern Med. 2015;162(3):205–213. [https://www.ncbi.nlm.nih.gov/pubmed/25383671]

▼ IMMUNE THROMBOCYTOPENIC PURPURA

Initial Assessment (ASH 2011)

1. Chronic acquired bleeding disorder: Autoantibodies against platelet antigens
2. Primary ITP: No known trigger
3. Secondary ITP: Caused by another disease, condition, or infection (infections, hypersplenism, alcohol, nutrient deficiency, autoimmune disorders, malignancy, other hematologic conditions)
4. Drug-induced ITP: Many drugs can cause ITP; perform a thorough medication reconciliation and review[6]
5. Diagnosis of exclusion
   a. Thrombocytopenia (platelet count $<150,000/\mu L$) with no other observable cause
   b. Perform a complete physical exam looking for:
      i. Signs of bleeding (especially purpura, petechiae, epistaxis, gum bleeding)
      ii. Hepatosplenomegaly
   c. Order peripheral blood smear, HIV, HCV, coagulation studies, thyroid studies, *H. pylori* testing; consider further studies guided by history and exam

---

[6]Heparin-induced thrombocytopenia (HIT) paradoxically is a hypercoagulable state and can lead to venous and arterial thrombosis.

Acute Medical Management (ASH 2011)

1. Do not concentrate solely on platelet count
2. Serious bleeding most often seen when platelet count <20,000/μL; admit these patients and obtain hematology consultation
3. Platelets <30,000/μL or any number of platelets with bleeding
   a. First, transfuse platelets to a goal of >20,000/μL
   b. Next, trial glucocorticoids; cheaper and more readily available than IVIG
      i. Preferred: Dexamethasone 40 mg orally daily for 3 days
      ii. Alternate: Prednisone 1 mg/kg orally daily for 1–2 weeks followed by a taper over 4–6 weeks
      iii. Expect an increase in platelet count within 2 weeks
   c. Third, start IVIG; raises platelets faster than glucocorticoids
      i. Ensure HIV/HCV negative
      ii. Ensure vaccinations status is up to date
      iii. Use 1 g/kg as a onetime dose
      iv. Expect an increase in platelet count in 24–48 hours
4. Platelets ≥30,000/μL: Observe
5. ITP in pregnancy
   a. 10× higher risk than in general population
   b. Workup and treatment is the same as the general population
      i. Transfusion if bleeding or <20,000/μL
      ii. Glucocorticoids
      iii. IVIG
      iv. Hematology consultation

Interventions (ASH 2011)

1. If platelet count remains <20,000/μL or bleeding continues
   a. Consult a general surgeon for possible splenectomy
   b. Consult a hematologist for other treatment modalities

Source:

1. ASH 2011: Neunert C, Lim W, Crowther M, et al. The American Society of Hematology 2011 evidence-based practice guideline for immune thrombocytopenia. Blood. 2011;117(16):4190–4207. [https://www.ncbi. nlm.nih.gov/pubmed/21325604]

THROMBOTIC THROMBOCYTOPENIC PURPURA

Initial Assessment (BCSH 2012)

1. Thrombotic thrombocytopenic purpura (TTP) is a medical emergency
2. Types
   a. Hereditary: Inherited mutations in ADAMST13
   b. Acquired: Deficiency of ADAMST13

3. Symptoms: Weakness, dizziness, petechiae, bleeding
4. Labs to order
   a. CBC: Thrombocytopenia and microangiopathic hemolytic anemia (MAHA)
   b. Peripheral blood smear
   c. Serum chemistries
   d. Creatinine
   e. LDH: Elevated
   f. Bilirubin: Elevated
   g. Haptoglobin
   h. Coagulation times (PT/PTT): Normal
   i. Fibrinogen
   j. D-dimer
   k. Direct antiglobulin test (DAT COOMBS): Negative
   l. ADAMTS13 activity and inhibitor testing

Acute Medical Management (BCSH 2012)

1. TTP is lethal; initiate treatment if clinically suspicious even before labs return; obtain hematology consultation stat
   a. Daily plasma exchange
      i. Consider plasma infusion if exchange is not readily available
      ii. Requires central venous catheter
   b. Glucocorticoids
      i. Prednisone 1 mg/kg per day
      ii. OR methylprednisolone 125 mg BID – q6 hours
   c. Expect increase in platelets in 48–72 hours

Source:

1. BCSH 2012: Scully M, Hunt BJ, Benjamin S, et al. Guidelines on the diagnosis and management of thrombotic thrombocytopenic purpura and other thrombotic microangiopathies. Br J Haematol. 2012;158(3):323–335. [https://www.ncbi.nlm.nih.gov/pubmed/22624596]

HEPARIN-INDUCED THROMBOCYTOPENIA

Initial Assessment (BCSH 2012)

1. Determine Pretest Probability of Heparin-Induced Thrombocytopenia (HIT) Using 4Ts Score (See Table 7-1)
   a. If 4Ts score is low (0–3), exclude HIT with no need for laboratory investigation
   b. If 4Ts score is intermediate (4–5), exclude HIT with a negative gel particle immunoassay
   c. If 4Ts score is high (6–8), run ELISA antigen assay for surface-bound PF4-heparin complexes

TABLE 7-1

4Ts SCORE FOR HIT PRETEST PROBABILITY			
	2 Points	**1 Point**	**0 Points**
Thrombocytopenia	>50% fall and platelet nadir $\geq$20 × 10^9/L	30%–50% fall or platelet nadir 10–19 × 10^9/L	Fall <30% or platelet nadir <10 × 10^9/L
Timing of platelet count fall or other sequelae	Clear onset between days 5 and 10[1] Or, $\leq$1 day (if heparin exposure within past 30 days)	Consistent with immunization but not clear (e.g., missing platelet counts) or onset of thrombocytopenia after day 10; or fall $\leq$1 day if heparin exposure was 30–100 days ago	Platelet count fall $\leq$4 days (without recent heparin exposure)
Thrombosis or other sequelae (e.g., skin lesions)	New thrombosis; skin necrosis; post-heparin bolus acute systemic reaction	Progressive or recurrent thrombosis; erythematous skin lesions; suspected thrombosis not yet proven	None
Other cause for thrombocytopenia not evident	No other cause for platelet count fall is evident	Possible other cause is evident	Definite other cause is present

[1]First day of immunizing heparin exposure is considered day 0. The first day the platelet count begins to fall is considered the day of onset of thrombocytopenia.
Source: Lo GK et al. J Thromb Haemost. 2006 Apr;4(4):759–65. Table 1.
Assign 0, 1, or 2 points for each of four categories. Maximum possible score is 8.
Pretest probability score: 6–8 = high, 4–5 = intermediate, 0–3 = low.

Acute Medical Management (BSCH 2012)
1. If the 4Ts score is not low (0–3), stop heparin immediately and start a full-dose alternative anticoagulant (e.g., danaparoid, fondaparinux, argatroban)
2. Do not use LMWH in HIT

Management After Stabilization (BCSH 2012)
1. Avoid warfarin until platelet count has returned to the normal range
2. When warfarin is started, continue alternative anticoagulant until INR is in the therapeutic range

3. Do not give platelets for prophylaxis; consider giving platelets in the event of bleeding
4. Therapeutic anticoagulation
   a. Give for 3 months after HIT with a thrombotic complication
   b. Give for 4 weeks after HIT without a thrombotic complication
5. Delay surgery in patients with recent or active HIT until patient is antibody-negative
6. If urgent surgery is required, use bivalirudin as alternative anticoagulant

Sources:

1. BCSH 2012: Watson, H, Davidson S, Keeling D. Guidelines on the diagnosis and management of heparin-induced thrombocytopenia: second edition. Br J Haematol. 2012;159(5):528–540. [https://www.ncbi.nlm.nih.gov/pubmed/23043677]
2. Lo GK, Juhl D, Warkentin TE, et al. Evaluation of pretest clinical score (4 T's) for the diagnosis of heparin-induced thrombocytopenia in two clinical settings. J Thromb Haemost. 2006 Apr;4(4):759–765. [https://www.ncbi.nlm.nih.gov/pubmed/16634744]

SICKLE CELL DISEASE: VASO-OCCLUSIVE CRISIS

Initial Assessment (NHLBI 2014)
1. Determine characteristics, location, and intensity of pain
2. Assess patient's recent analgesic use (opioid and nonopioid)

Acute Medical Management (NHLBI 2014)
1. Initiate analgesics within 30 minutes of triage or 60 minutes of registration
2. Base analgesic selection on pain assessment, associated symptoms, outpatient analgesic use, patient knowledge of effective agents and doses, and history of side effects
3. If patient has mild-to-moderate pain and reports relief with NSAIDs, continue NSAID treatment (in the absence of contraindications)
4. If patient has severe pain, rapidly initiate treatment with parenteral opioids
5. Administer subcutaneous opioids if IV access is difficult
6. Reassess pain and readminister opioids if necessary for continued severe pain every 15–30 minutes
7. Consider dose escalation by 25% until pain is controlled

Management After Stabilization (NHLBI 2014)
1. Initiate around-the-clock opioid administration by PCA, frequently scheduled doses, or PRN doses
2. If PCA does not have a basal rate, continue long-acting oral opioids
3. If PCA does have a basal rate, consider stopping long-acting oral opioids to prevent oversedation

4. Continue to use oral NSAIDs as an adjuvant analgesic in the absence of contraindications
5. Do not use meperidine unless it is the only effective opioid for a patient
6. Encourage incentive spirometry, activity, and ambulation to reduce risk of acute chest syndrome
7. Administer supplemental oxygen for patients with an oxygen saturation <95%
8. In patients who are euvolemic but unable to drink fluids, provide IV hydration at no more than maintenance rate to avoid overhydration
9. At discharge: Evaluate inpatient analgesic requirements, wean parental opioids prior to conversion to oral opioids, and adjust home doses of opioids to prevent withdrawal after discharge

Source:
1. NHLBI 2014: Yawn BP, Buchanan GR, Afenyi-Annan AN, et al. Evidence-based management of sickle cell disease: expert panel report, 2014. JAMA. 2014;312(10):1033–1048. [https://www.ncbi.nlm.nih.gov/pubmed/25203083]

SICKLE CELL DISEASE: ACUTE CHEST SYNDROME

Initial Assessment (NHLBI 2014)
1. Suspect in patients with sickle cell disease (SCD) who develop acute onset of cough, shortness of breath, tachypnea, retractions, or wheezing with or without fever
2. Obtain chest X-ray and measure oxygen saturation

Acute Medical Management (NHLBI 2014)
1. Initiate antibiotic therapy with an IV cephalosporin and PO macrolide
2. Use supplemental oxygen to maintain oxygen saturation >95% if patient has mild-to-moderate pain and reports relief with NSAIDs, continue NSAID treatment (in the absence of contraindications)

Interventions (NHLBI 2014)
1. In patients with symptomatic ACS whose hemoglobin is >1.0 g/dL below baseline, give simple blood transfusion (10 mL/kg red blood cells) to improve oxygen-carrying capacity (may not be required if baseline hemoglobin is 9.0 g/dL or higher)
2. In patients with HbSC disease or HbSβ+-thalassemia, consult an SCD expert prior to transfusion
3. When there is rapid progression of ACS (manifested by oxygen saturation below 90% despite supplemental oxygen, increasing respiratory distress, progressive pulmonary infiltrates, and/or decline in hemoglobin concentration despite simple transfusion), perform urgent exchange

transfusion (consult hematology, critical care, and/or apheresis specialists)

Management After Stabilization (NHLBI 2014)

1. Monitor closely for bronchospasm, acute anemia, hypoxemia
2. Incentive spirometry while awake

Source:

1. NHLBI 2014: Yawn BP, Buchanan GR, Afenyi-Annan AN, et al. Evidence-based management of sickle cell disease: expert panel report, 2014. JAMA. 2014;312(10):1033–1048. [https://www.ncbi.nlm.nih.gov/pubmed/25203083]

Renal

Kristi M. Schoeld

ACUTE KIDNEY INJURY

Initial Assessment

1. Assessing risk and preventing acute kidney injury (AKI) (see page 191)
2. Definition and staging (KDIGO 2012)
   a. AKI is defined as any of the following:
      i. Increase in serum Cr by ≥0.3 mg/dL within 48 hours; or
      ii. Increase in serum Cr to ≥1.5× baseline within 7 days; or
      iii. Urine volume <0.5 mL/kg/h for 6 hours
   b. AKI is staged for severity
      i. Stage 1: Cr 1.5–1.9× baseline or ≥0.3 mg/dL increase; UOP <0.5 mL/kg/h for 6–12 hours
      ii. Stage 2: Cr 2.0–2.9× baseline; UOP <0.5 mL/kg/h for ≥12 hours
      iii. Stage 3: Cr 3.0× baseline or Cr ≥4.0 mg/dL or dialysis; UOP <0.3 mL/kg/h for ≥24 hours or anuria for ≥12 hours
3. Identify the cause of AKI (NCGC 2013)
   a. Obtain urinalysis
      i. Dipstick UA for blood, protein, leukocytes, nitrites and glucose in all patients with AKI; document results and ensure appropriate action if abnormal
      ii. Consider acute nephritis and consult nephrology when a patient with AKI with no obvious cause has a urine dipstick showing protein or blood in the absence of UTI, menses, or trauma due to catheterization
   b. Obtain US if the cause of AKI is unknown
      i. When pyonephrosis is suspected, get an immediate US (within 6 hours)
      ii. With no identified cause of AKI, get an urgent US (within 24 hours)

Acute Medical Management

1. Relieve obstruction (NCGC 2013)
   a. When nephrostomy or stenting is used, undertake within 12 hours of diagnosis
   b. Immediate referral to urology for:
      i. Pyonephrosis
      ii. Obstructed solitary kidney
      iii. Bilateral hydronephrosis or bilateral ureteral obstruction
      iv. Complications of AKI caused by urological obstruction
2. Pharmacological management (NCGC 2013, KDIGO 2012)
   a. Loop diuretics
      i. Do not routinely use to treat AKI
      ii. Consider for treating fluid overload or edema while awaiting dialysis or while renal function is recovering if not on dialysis
   b. Fluids: Unless in shock, use isotonic crystalloids rather than colloids as initial management for volume expansion
   c. If vasomotor shock and AKI: Use vasopressors with fluids
   d. Do not use the following to treat AKI:
      i. Dopamine
      ii. Fenoldopam
      iii. ANP (atrial natriuretic peptide)
      iv. Recombinant human insulin-like growth hormone
   e. Anticoagulation in patients with AKI on dialysis
      i. Use anticoagulation during dialysis in AKI if the patient does not have an increased risk of bleeding or impaired coagulation and is not already receiving systemic anticoagulation
         1. Use unfractionated or low-molecular-weight (LMW) heparin for intermittent dialysis
         2. Use regional citrate anticoagulation for continuous dialysis; for patients on continuous dialysis with contraindications to citrate, use unfractionated or LMW heparin
      ii. For patients with increased risk of bleeding who are not on systemic anticoagulation:
         1. Use regional citrate during continuous dialysis in patients without contraindication for citrate
         2. Avoid regional heparin during continuous dialysis
      iii. For patients with HIT (heparin-induced thrombocytopenia):
         1. Use direct thrombin inhibitors (i.e., argatroban) or factor Xa inhibitors (i.e., fondaparinux) rather than other or no anticoagulation during dialysis
         2. In a patient with HIT and AKI on dialysis who does NOT have severe liver failure, use argatroban preferentially

Interventions

1. Refer to nephrology (NCGC 2013)
   a. Refer patients with AKI immediately if they meet criteria for dialysis
   b. Do not refer when there is a clear cause for AKI and the condition is responding promptly to treatment, unless they have a renal transplant
   c. Discuss the management of AKI with a nephrologist within 24 hours of detection of AKI when one or more of the following is present:
      i. Possible diagnosis that may need specialist treatment (i.e., vasculitis, glomerulonephritis, myeloma, etc.)
      ii. AKI with no clear cause
      iii. Inadequate response to treatment
      iv. Complications associated with AKI
      v. Stage 3 AKI
      vi. Renal transplant
      vii. CKD stage 4 or 5
2. Referring for renal replacement therapy (dialysis) (NCGC 2013, KDIGO 2012)
   a. Discuss potential indications for dialysis with nephrology immediately to ensure therapy is started as soon as needed
   b. When a patient has significant comorbidities, use shared decision making as to whether dialysis would offer benefit
   c. Refer for immediate dialysis if any of the following are not responding to medical management:
      i. Hyperkalemia
      ii. Metabolic acidosis
      iii. Symptoms or complications of uremia (i.e., pericarditis or encephalopathy)
      iv. Fluid overload
      v. Pulmonary edema
   d. Vascular access for dialysis
      i. Initiate dialysis with an uncuffed nontunneled dialysis catheter
      ii. Choice of veins
         1. First: Right jugular
         2. Second: Femoral
         3. Third: Left jugular
         4. Last choice: Subclavian with preference for dominant side
      iii. Use US guidance for dialysis catheter insertion
      iv. Get a CXR promptly after placement and before using an internal jugular or subclavian dialysis catheter
      v. Do not use topical antibiotics over the skin insertion site of a nontunneled catheter in ICU patients with AKI requiring dialysis
      vi. Do not use antibiotic locks for prevention of catheter-associated infections of nontunneled catheters in AKI requiring dialysis

e. Choice of continuous vs. standard intermittent dialysis
  i. Use continuous dialysis for hemodynamically unstable patients
  ii. Use continuous dialysis for AKI patients with acute brain injury or other causes of increased intracranial pressure or brain edema

Sources:

1. NCGC 2013: National Clinical Guideline Centre. Acute kidney injury. Prevention, detection and management of acute kidney injury up to the point of renal replacement therapy. London (UK): National Institute for Health and Care Excellence (NICE); 2013 Aug. 39 p. (Clinical guideline; no. 169). [https://www.guideline.gov/summaries/summary/47080]

2. KDIGO 2012: KDIGO clinical practice guideline for acute kidney injury. Kidney Int Suppl. 2012 Mar;2(Suppl 1):1–138. [http://kdigo.org/guidelines/acute-kidney-injury/]

Endocrine

9

Kristi M. Schoeld
Paul Opare-Addo

HYPOTHYROIDISM

Initial Assessment (CPGH 2012)

1. Only measure TSH in hospitalized patients if thyroid dysfunction suspected; in addition to measuring TSH:
   a. Obtain serum free T4 instead of total T4
   b. Do not measure total T3 or free T3
   c. In patients with central hypothyroidism, assess free T4 or free T4 index, not TSH, to diagnose and guide treatment
2. Anti-thyroid antibody testing
   a. Consider anti-thyroid peroxidase antibody (TPOAb) in subclinical hypothyroidism
   b. Consider TPOAb to identify autoimmune thyroiditis when nodular thyroid disease is suspected to be autoimmune
3. How to determine upper limit normal (ULN) for TSH
   a. Reference range changes with age; if an age-based ULN is not available in an iodine-sufficient area, use an ULN 4.12
4. In patients with TSH levels above lab reference range
   a. Patients with serum TSH >10 have increased risk of heart failure and cardiovascular mortality; give thyroid replacement
   b. Patients with serum TSH between ULN and 10: Individualize treatment based on symptoms suggestive of hypothyroidism, positive TPOAb, or evidence of ASCVD or heart failure or risk factors for these

Acute Medical Management (CPGH 2012)

1. Use L-thyroxine (T4) monotherapy
   a. Do not use combination T4 and T3 (L-triiodothyronine)
   b. Do not use dessiccated thyroid hormone
   c. Do not use TRIAC (tiratricol; 3,5,3-triiodothyroacetic acid) to treat primary or central hypothyroidism due to suggestion of harm

2. Dosing L-thyroxine
   a. Patients resuming therapy after interruption less than 6 weeks and without intercurrent cardiac event or marked weight loss may resume their previous full replacement dose
   b. When initiating therapy in young healthy adults with overt hypothyroidism begin with full replacement doses
   c. When initiating therapy in patients older than 50–60 with overt hypothyroidism, without CAD, start 50 mcg daily
   d. In patients with subclinical hypothyroidism, start 25–75 mcg daily depending on the degree of TSH elevation
3. Timing L-thyroxine therapy
   a. Take L-thyroxine with water 30–60 minutes before breakfast OR at bedtime 4 hours after the last meal
   b. Treat patients with combined adrenal insufficiency and hypothyroidism with glucocorticoids before starting L-thyroxine
4. Who not to treat
   a. Do not treat with thyroid hormones empirically without lab confirmation
   b. Do not treat obesity with thyroid hormones if euthyroid
   c. Do not treat depression with thyroid hormones if euthyroid
5. Consider endocrine consult if:
   a. Patients difficult to render and maintain euthyroid state
   b. Hypothyroid patients with cardiac disease
   c. Hypothyroid patients with goiter, nodule, or structural changes to gland
   d. Hypothyroid patients with other endocrine diseases, i.e., adrenal or pituitary
   e. Unusual constellation of thyroid test results
   f. Unusual causes of hypothyroidism, i.e., central or secondary causes

Management After Stabilization (CPGH 2012)
1. Patients being treated with established hypothyroidism
   a. Measure TSH 4–8 weeks after initiating therapy or changing doses; once therapeutic, measure TSH at 6- and then 12-month intervals or when clinically indicated
   b. Remeasure TSH within 4–8 weeks of initiation of treatment with drugs that decrease the bioavailability or alter the metabolic distribution of L-thyroxine
   c. Consider checking serum free T4 with TSH
2. Determining target TSH
   a. In nonpregnant patients, goal of therapy is a TSH WNL; if reference ranges are not available, use range 0.45–4.12
   b. In nonpregnant patients, the evidence does not support targeting specific TSH values within normal range

Source:

1. CPGH 2012: Garber JR, Cobin RH, Gharib H, et al. American Association of Clinical Endocrinologists and American Thyroid Association. Clinical practice guidelines for hypothyroidism in adults: cosponsored by the American Association of Clinical Endocrinologists and the American Thyroid Association. Endocr Pract. 2012;18(6):988–1028. [http://guideline.gov/summaries/summary/46419?#420]

HYPERTHYROIDISM

Initial Assessment (ATA/AACE 2011)
1. Measure a TSH and free T4 and either total or free T3
2. Do a radioactive iodine uptake when the presentation of thyrotoxicosis is not diagnostic of Graves' disease (GD)[1]
   a. Normal or elevated uptake seen in GD, toxic multinodular goiter (TMNG) or toxic adenoma (TA), and TSH producing pituitary adenomas
   b. Near-absent uptake seen in acute and subacute thyroiditis, amiodarone-induced thyroiditis, iatrogenic thyrotoxicosis, factitious ingestion of thyroid hormone, and extensive metastasis from follicular thyroid cancer
3. Do a thyroid US if there are thyroid nodules
4. Assess for disease severity: Check for cardiac, ophtho, and CNS manifestations of thyroid disease, as well as GI and thermoregulatory dysfunction

Acute Medical Management (ATA/AACE 2011)
1. Symptomatic management
   a. Give beta blockers to elderly patients with symptoms and to other thyrotoxic patients with resting HR >90 or coexistent heart disease
   b. Consider beta blockers in all patients with symptomatic disease
   c. Propranolol, atenolol, metoprolol, nadolol, or esmolol can be used
2. Thyroid Storm (See Table 9-1 for Diagnostic Criteria): Multimodal Treatment Including
   a. Beta blockers (propranolol 60–80 mg every 4 hours)
   b. Anti-thyroid drugs (ATD): PTU 500–1000 mg load, then 250 mg every 6 hours, or methimazole 60–80 mg/day
   c. Inorganic iodine (SSKI) – Start 1 hour after ATDs, 5 drops (0.25 mL or 250 mg) orally every 6 hours
   d. Corticosteroid therapy (hydrocortisone 300 mg IV load, then 100 mg every 8 hours)

[1] In a patient with symmetrically enlarged thyroid, recent onset of ophthalmopathy, and moderate-to-severe hyperthyroidism, the diagnosis of GD is sufficiently likely that further evaluation is unnecessary.

TABLE 9-1

POINT SCALE FOR THE DIAGNOSIS OF THYROID STORM

Scores >45 consistent with thyroid storm, 25–44 impending thyroid storm, <25 storm unlikely (Burch 1993)

Temperature

99.0–99.9	5 pts
100.0–100.9	10 pts
101.0–101.9	15 pts
102.0–102.9	20 pts
103.0–103.9	25 pts
≥104	30 pts

Pulse

100–109	5 pts
110–119	10 pts
120–129	15 pts
130–139	20 pts
≥140	25 pts

Atrial fibrillation

Absent	0 pts
Present	10 pts

CHF

Absent	0 pts
Mild	5 pts
Moderate	10 pts
Severe	20 pts

GI/Hepatic dysfunction

Absent	0 pts
Moderate (diarrhea, abdominal pain, nausea/vomiting)	10 pts
Severe (jaundice)	20 pts

CNS disturbance

Absent	0 pts
Mild (agitation)	10 pts
Moderate (delirium, psychosis, extreme lethargy)	20 pts
Severe (seizure, coma)	30 pts

(Continued)

TABLE 9-1 (*Continued*)

POINT SCALE FOR THE DIAGNOSIS OF THYROID STORM

Precipitant history (i.e., abrupt cessation of anti-thyroid drug, surgery in the setting of inadequately treated thyrotoxicosis)

Positive	0 pts
Negative	10 pts

Source: Nayak B, Burman K. Thyrotoxicosis and thyroid storm. Endocrinol Metab Clin North Am. 2006 Dec;35(4): 663–86, vii, Tab 1.

    e. Aggressive cooling with acetaminophen and cooling blankets
    f. Volume resuscitation
    g. Respiratory support and monitoring in an ICU
  3. Treat GD with any of the following:
    a. Radioactive iodine: Favored in females planning future pregnancy, patients at high surgical risk, patients with history of neck surgery or irradiation, lack of access to high-volume thyroid surgeon, or contraindications to ATD use
      i. Pretreat with beta blockers if extremely symptomatic or free T4 2–3× ULN
      ii. Consider pretreatment with methimazole for patients who are extremely symptomatic or have free T4 2–3× ULN
      iii. Medically optimize comorbid conditions before giving radioactive iodine
      iv. Obtain pregnancy test within 48 hours prior to treatment
      v. Give sufficient radiation in a single dose to render the patient hypothyroid
    b. ATDs: Favored in the elderly or others with comorbidities increasing surgical risk or limiting life expectancy, those with moderate-to-severe active Graves' ophthalmopathy (GO), patients with history of neck surgery or radiation, or if there is no access to high-volume thyroid surgeon
      i. Use methimazole in virtually every patient except during first trimester pregnancy and for thyroid storm
      ii. Get a baseline CBC with differential (CBCD) and liver profile before starting therapy
    c. Thyroidectomy/surgery: Favored with symptomatic compression or large goiters, concern for malignancy, coexisting hyperparathyroidism requiring surgery, patients with moderate-or-severe active GO, and females planning to be pregnant soon
      i. When possible, render patients with GD euthyroid with methimazole pre-operative
      ii. If unable to render a GD patient euthyroid pre-op, treat with beta blockers immediately pre-op

      iii. Give potassium iodide (SSKI) immediately pre-op

      iv. Near total or total thyroidectomy is the procedure of choice, preferably done by high-volume thyroid surgeon

      v. Stop ATDs at the time of surgery

   4. TMNG or TA: Treat with the following:

     a. Radioactive iodine (iodine 131)

       i. Treat with beta blockers prior to starting therapy if increased risk for complications (elderly, heart disease, or severe hyperthyroidism); continue until euthyroid state is achieved

       ii. Consider pretreatment with methimazole prior to starting therapy in patients at increased risk for complications

       iii. Give sufficient radiation in a single dose to alleviate hyperthyroidism

     b. Surgery

       i. Render patients euthyroid with methimazole before surgery, with or without beta blocker therapy

       ii. Do not use pre-op iodine

       iii. For TMNG, perform near-total or total thyroidectomy

       iv. For TA, perform an ipsilateral thyroid lobectomy, or isthmusectomy if the adenoma is in the isthmus

       v. Stop methimazole at the time of surgery

     c. Avoid ATDs for treatment of TMNG or TA

   5. Thyroid nodules, whether euthyroid or in GD

     a. Evaluate nodules >1–1.5 cm size before radioactive iodine therapy

     b. If a radioactive iodine scan is performed, consider FNA of nonfunctioning or hypofunctioning ("cold") nodules

     c. If cytopathology is suspicious or diagnostic of malignancy, surgery is advised after normalization of thyroid function with ATDs (if not already euthyroid)

   6. GO[2]: Quickly achieve and maintain euthyroid state

     a. Advise all to quit smoking

     b. In patients with mild active GO who are nonsmokers, either radioactive iodine, methimazole, or thyroidectomy are equally acceptable therapies

     c. If radioactive iodine is chosen, consider concurrent treatment with corticosteroids

     d. Give corticosteroids concurrently to patients with mild active GO who are smokers, and who choose radioactive iodine

     e. Offer methimazole or surgery (not radioactive iodine) to patients with moderate-to-severe active GO

---

[2]Graves' ophthalmopathy severity assessment depends on lid retraction (< or >2 mm), degree of soft tissue involvement (mild, moderate, or severe), proptosis (< or >3 mm), diplopia (absent, transient, or constant), corneal exposure (absent, mild, severe), or optic nerve status (normal or compression). It is graded as mild, moderate, severe, or sight threatening.

7. Drug-induced thyrotoxicosis
   a. Iodine-induced hyperthyroidism: Use beta blockers alone or in combo with methimazole
   b. Cytokine-induced thyrotoxicosis: Evaluate patients on alpha interferon or interleukin 2 therapy who develop thyrotoxicosis to determine etiology (painless thyroiditis vs. GD) and treat accordingly
   c. Amiodarone-induced thyrotoxicosis (AIT)
      i. Classification
         1. Type 1 is iodine-induced
         2. Type 2 is a destructive thyroiditis
         3. Consider testing to distinguish which type is present, but the distinction between the two types is not always clear and some patients have elements of both[3]
      ii. Treatment
         1. Use methimazole for type 1
         2. Use corticosteroids for type 2
         3. Use both methimazole and corticosteroids in patients who fail to respond to single modality therapy and in patients in whom type is unequivocally determined
         4. Offer thyroidectomy to patients who fail to respond to dual drug therapy
         5. Make the decision to stop amiodarone in consultation with a cardiologist, based on the availability of effective alternative antiarrhythmic therapy
8. Destructive thyroiditis (includes postpartum, painless, subacute, acute, traumatic, and drug-induced)
   a. Subacute thyroiditis
      i. Mild symptomatic: Give beta blockers and NSAIDs
      ii. Moderate-to-severe symptoms, or failure to respond: Give corticosteroids

Management After Stabilization (ATA/AACE 2011)

1. Graves' disease
   a. On ATDs
      i. With any febrile illness or pharyngitis, recheck CBCD
      ii. With any pruritic rash, jaundice, joint pain, abdominal pain, anorexia, nausea or vomiting – recheck liver profile
      iii. For minor allergic cutaneous reactions, add antihistamine therapy; with persistent minor reactions, change ATD or choice of therapy; for severe allergic reactions, stop ATDs and change therapy

---

[3]RAIU is occasionally measurable in type 1 AIT but not type 2 AIT, increased vascular flow on color-flow Doppler US may be seen in type 1 AIT but not type 2 AIT. Measurement of serum interleukin-6 levels does not reliably distinguish between the two types of AIT.

    b. Status post thyroidectomy

        i. Check serum calcium (6 and 12 hours post-op) or PTH intact and consider oral calcium and calcitriol supplementation as needed

        ii. Wean beta blockers following surgery

        iii. Give post-op L-thyroxine dosed by weight (1.7 mcg/kg or 0.8 mcg/lb)

2. TMNG or TA

    a. Status post thyroidectomy

        i. Check serum calcium (6 and 12 hours post-op) or PTH intact and consider oral calcium and calcitriol supplementation as needed

        ii. Slowly wean beta blockers following surgery

        iii. Give post-op L-thyroxine dosed by weight (1.7 mcg/kg or 0.8 mcg/lb)

        iv. Use radioactive iodine for retreatment or persistent hyperthyroidism following surgery

Sources:

1. ATA/AACE Guidelines 2011: Bahn RS, Burch HB, Cooper DS, et al. Hyperthyroidism and other causes of thyrotoxicosis: management guidelines of the American Thyroid Association and American Association of Clinical Endocrinologists. Endocr Pract. 2011;17(3):456–520. [https://www.ncbi.nlm.nih.gov/pubmed/21700562]

2. Burch HB, Wartofsky L. Life-threatening thyrotoxicosis. Thyroid storm. Endocrinol Metab Clin North Am. 1993 Jun;22(2):263–277. [https://www.ncbi.nlm.nih.gov/pubmed/8325286]

HYPERGLYCEMIA

Initial Assessment (AACE/ACE 2011, AACE/ADA 2009, ADA 2016, ES 2012)

1. Draw A1c, CBC

Acute Medical Management

1. Critical care

    a. Insulin[4] (AACE/ADA 2009)

        i. Use IV insulin infusion with frequent glucose monitoring to prevent hypoglycemia

    b. Glucose goals (ADA 2016, AACE/ACE 2015, ACP 2011)

        i. Blood glucose goals are 140–180 mg/dL[5] (7.8–10 mmol/L) even if in ICU[6]; increased risk of mortality with hypoglycemia starting from <140 mg/dL

---

[4] AACE/ACE 2015, AACE/ADA 2009 – Noninsulin antihyperglycemic agents not appropriate.

[5] ACP 2011 – Recommends 140–200 mg/dL.

[6] No benefit to stricter/tighter blood (80–110 mg/dL) sugar control in the short term, although may be applicable in certain individuals. Avoid hypoglycemia. And higher glucose levels may be acceptable in terminal ill individuals.

      ii. AACE/ADA 2009, ADA 2016: If persistent hyperglycemia, start insulin therapy at 180 mg/dL

  c. Hypoglycemia[7]

      i. Avoid hypoglycemia

2. Noncritical care

  a. Insulin/Glucose goals

      i. AACE/ACE 2015: Fasting <140 mg/dL and random <180 mg/dL

      ii. ADA 2016: 140–180 mg/dL (7.8–10.0 mmol/L)

Interventions

1. Perioperative management for critical/noncritical care

  a. ADA 2016: Perioperative target glucose range: 80–180 mg/dL

  b. ES 2012: Infuse insulin or give subcutaneous basal insulin with bolus as required perioperatively

Management After Stabilization

1. Critical care

  a. Insulin (ADA 2016, AACE/ADA 2009)

      i. Use scheduled subcutaneous insulin consisting of a basal, a nutritional, and supplemental/correction

      ii. Do not use only sliding scale insulin regimen

      iii. Make changes based on daily patterns, paying attention to transitions (diet status/caloric intake)

  b. Glucose goals (AACE/ACE 2015)

      i. Remain the same

  c. Medical nutrition therapy calorie goals (AACE/ACE 2015)

      i. 15–25 calories/kg/day[8]

      ii. Include Certified Diabetes Educators in care of patient

  d. Discharge (ADA 2016, AACE/ACE 2015, AACE/ADA 2009)

      i. Start discharge planning at time of admission

      ii. Prepare a clear plan for follow-up and close monitoring

      iii. Communicate with outpatient provider

2. Noncritical care

  a. Insulin (ADA 2016, AACE/ACE 2015, ES 2012)

      i. Use insulin therapy only; discontinue all oral hypoglycemics

      ii. Use scheduled subcutaneous insulin consisting of a basal, a nutritional, and supplemental/correction

      iii. Taking PO: Give subcutaneous insulin injections to align with meals and bedtime; give basal, nutritional, and correction components

---

[7]Defined as blood glucose <70 mg/dL and severe hypoglycemia as <40 mg/dL.
[8]AACE/ACE – Equivalent to 1800–2000 calories/day or 200 g carbohydrate per day. This encompasses meals and snacks. The ADA does not endorse any specific meal plan.

     iv. NPO or on enteral/parenteral therapy: Give subcutaneous insulin injections every 4–6 hours

     v. NPO or has poor PO intake: Give short-acting insulin post meals

     vi. ES 2012, ADA 2010: If patient has diabetes (T1 or T2) and transitioning from infusion, give subcutaneous insulin 1–2 hours before stopping continuous infusion

     vii. ES 2012: Start scheduled insulin therapy if blood sugar >140 mg/dL regardless of diabetes history if requiring 12–24 hours of insulin for sugar correction

     viii. ES 2012/ADA 2010: If receiving therapies causing hyperglycemia such as enteral or peripheral nutrition, steroid or octreotide, regardless of DM history, continue POC testing for 24–48 hours

     ix. ES 2012: If patient is receiving steroids and blood sugar >140 mg/dL, regardless of diabetes status, start insulin therapy

     x. ES 2012: Start insulin drip if unable to control blood sugars with subcutaneous insulin

     xi. ES 2012: Stop POC testing if no DM and no requirement of insulin for 24–48 hours if patient is at appropriate caloric intake

  b. Glucose goals (ES 2012)

     i. Fasting goals of <140 mg/dL and random goal of <180 mg/dL[9]

     ii. If no history of diabetes, but with blood glucose >140 mg/dL, monitor via POC testing for at least 24–48 hours

     iii. POC testing every 4–6 hours for NPO patients; otherwise POC testing before meals and at bedtime

     iv. Reassess antidiabetic therapy if 100 mg/dL blood sugar or less

  c. Medical nutrition therapy (AACE/ACE 2015, AACE/ADA 2009, ES 2012)

     i. Goal 25–35 calories/kg/day; consistent carbohydrate amount for meals

  d. Discharge (ES 2012)

     i. Restart preadmission diabetes regimen (insulin or non-insulin/orals)

     ii. Start insulin no less than 24 hours prior to discharge to assess efficacy

     iii. Otherwise, as above

Sources:

1. ADA 2010: American Diabetes Association. Standards of medical care in diabetes – 2010. Diabetes Care. 2010;33(Suppl 1):S11–S61. [http://care.diabetesjournals.org/content/33/Supplement_1/S11]

2. ADA 2016: American Diabetes Association. 13. Diabetes care in the hospital. Diabetes Care. 2016;39(Suppl 1):S99–S104. [http://care.diabetesjournals.org/content/39/Supplement_1/S99]

3. AACE/ACE 2015: Handelsman Y, Bloomgarden ZT, Grunberger G, et al. American Association of Clinical Endocrinologists and American College

---

[9]ADA 2010 – Agreed on by the American Diabetes Association.

of Endocrinology – clinical practice guidelines for developing a diabetes mellitus comprehensive care plan – 2015. Endocr Pract. 2015;21(Suppl 1): 1–87. [https://www.aace.com/publications/guidelines]

4. ACP 2011: Qaseem A, Humphrey LL, Chou R, Clinical Guidelines Committee of the American College of Physicians. Use of intensive insulin therapy for the management of glycemic control in hospitalized patients: a clinical practice guideline from the American College of Physicians. Ann Intern Med. 2011;154(4):260–267. [http://annals.org/aim/article/746815/use-intensive-insulin-therapy-management-glycemic-control-hospitalized-patients-clinical]

5. AACE/ADA 2009: Moghissi ES, Korytkowski MT, DiNardo M, et al. American Association of Clinical Endocrinologists and American Diabetes Association consensus statement on inpatient glycemic control. Diabetes Care. 2009;32(6):1119–1131. [https://www.aace.com/files/inpatientglycemiccontrolconsensusstatement.pdf]

6. ADA 2013: American Diabetes Association – diagnosis and classification of diabetes Mellitus. Diabetes Care. 2013;36(Suppl 1):S67–S74. [http://care.diabetesjournals.org/content/36/Supplement_1/S67]

7. ES 2012: Umpierrez GE, Hellman R, Korytkowski MT, et al. Management of hyperglycemia in hospitalized patients in non-critical care setting: an endocrine society clinical practice guideline. J Clin Endocrinol Metab. 2012;97(1):16–38. [https://www.guideline.gov/summaries/summary/35255?]

8. ADA 2009: Kitabchi AE, Umpierrez GE, Miles JM, Fisher JN. Hyperglycemic crises in adult patients with diabetes. Diabetes Care. 2009;32(7):1335–1343. [http://care.diabetesjournals.org/content/32/7/1335]

9. AAFP 2013: Westerberg DP. Diabetic ketoacidosis: evaluation and treatment. Am Fam Physician. 2013;87(5):337–346. [http://www.aafp.org/afp/2013/0301/p337.html]

HYPERGLYCEMIC CRISIS: DIABETIC KETOACIDOSIS AND HYPEROSMOLAR HYPERGLYCEMIC SYNDROME

Initial Assessment

1. History (ADA 2009, AAFP 2013)
   a. Get appropriate history including drug abuse, polyuria, polydipsia, weight loss, vomiting, dehydration, weakness, and mental status change
2. Physical exam (ADA 2009, AAFP 2013)
   a. Monitor for the following signs:
      i. DKA: Kussmaul breathing, N/V, abdominal pain
      ii. HHS: Lethargy/coma; focal neurologic signs, seizures
   b. Monitor temperature; severe hypothermia is a poor prognostic sign

3. Labs (ADA 2009, AAFP 2013)
   a. Arterial pH, serum bicarb, urine ketone, serum ketone,[10] serum osmolality, anion gap, plasma glucose, BUN, Cr, electrolyte
   b. CMP[11]; CBCD[12]; assess accurate Na levels by adding 1.6 mg/dL to measured Na for every 100 mg/dL of glucose above 100 mg/dL
   c. Get urine toxicology,[13] serum ethanol, and salicylate levels to rule out other causes of osmolar anion gap
   d. Post-diagnosis labs/imaging – Get CXR, urine, sputum, and blood cultures
   e. Assess mental status; if any changes (stupor, coma) without increase in osmolality, look for other causes of mental status change
4. Diagnostic criteria (ADA 2009)
   a. DKA: Blood glucose 250 mg/dL, arterial pH 7.3, bicarbonate 15 mEq/L, and moderate ketonuria or ketonemia
   b. HHS: Serum glucose >600 mEq/dL, arterial pH >7.3, serum bicarbonate >15 mEq/L, and minimal ketonemia

Acute Medical Management (ADA 2009, AAFP 2013)

1. General approach
   a. Treat precipitating factor[14]
   b. Get an EKG to assess for arrhythmias; if low or normal K, replete
   c. Further evaluate for other causes of abdominal pain,[15] if the pain is persistent with resolution of dehydration and metabolic acidosis[16]
2. Fluid therapy
   a. Infuse isotonic saline at 15–20 mL/kg/h or 1–1.5 L in the first hour
   b. Then infuse 0.45% NaCl at 250–500 mL/h (4–14 mL/kg/h) if corrected Na is normal or elevated[17]; otherwise 0.9% NaCl if corrected Na is low
   c. Monitor labs, urine output, hemodynamics, state of hydration, and physical exam to determine adequacy of rehydration[18]
   d. Avoid iatrogenic fluid overload in renal and cardiac patients
3. Insulin therapy
   a. Give continuous insulin therapy until resolution of crisis[19]

[10] ADA 2009 – More diagnostic for DKA.
[11] ADA 2009 – Normal or increased Na means severe water loss.
[12] ADA 2009/AAFP 2013 – Leukocytosis with cell counts >25 may mean infection. Bandemia is more predictive of infection.
[13] ADA 2009 – Cocaine can precipitate DKA.
[14] ADA 2009 – Most common is infection. Others are suboptimal therapy, non-adherence, MI, CVA.
[15] ADA 2009/AAFP 2013 – DKA can coexist with pancreatitis.
[16] AAFP 2013 – Anion gap >16 mEq/L.
[17] AAFP 2013 – >135 mEq/L.
[18] ADA 2009 – Goal is to correct fluid deficit within the first 24 hours. Aggressive rehydration is recommended.
[19] ADA 2009 – Ketoacidosis (blood glucose <200 mg/dL and two of the following: bicarb ≥15 mEq/L, venous pH >7.3, and a calculated anion gap ≤12 mEq/L. NB AAFP recommends >18 mEq/L; HHS (osmolality and regain of mental status).

    b. Infuse IV insulin[20] at 0.14 U/kg[21]; increase rate if not achieving 50–75 mg/dL/h decrease in blood sugar

    c. Decrease rate to 0.02–0.05 U/kg/h if blood sugar is 200 mg/dL in DKA or 300 mg/dL in HHS

    d. Add 5% dextrose when reducing infusion rate

    e. Transition from continuous to subcutaneous insulin as discussed above under hyperglycemia; do not transition if patient is NPO

4. Electrolyte repletion[22]

    a. Start K replacement at 10–15 mEq/h if K levels are within normal range; if <3.3 mEq/L, start at 20–30 mEq/h; goal is to keep levels at 4–5 mEq/L

    b. If patient is in DKA and hypokalemic, replete K to >3.3 mEq/L prior to insulin infusion[23]

    c. If pH <6.9, give 100 mEq sodium bicarbonate (2 amp) in 400 mL sterile water (isotonic solution) with 20 mEq KCl at a rate of 200 mL/h for 2 hours until venous pH is >7.0; if necessary, repeat every 2 hours until pH >7.0[24]

    d. In DKA, replace phosphate if any of the following: Cardiac dysfunction, anemia, respiratory depression, or phosphate levels <1.0 mEq/dL, or symptoms of hypophosphatemia[25]

    e. Replete Mg if it falls <1.2 mg/dL or if develops symptoms of hypomagnesemia[26]

5. Complications

    a. Monitor for signs of cerebral edema, including headaches, persistent vomiting, HTN, bradycardia, lethargy, and neurologic changes

6. Management algorithm: See Figure 9-1

Management After Stabilization (ADA 2009, AAFP 2013)

1. Put established diabetics on home regimen with changes to optimize clinical needs

2. Otherwise, as discussed above (see section "Hyperglycemia")

Sources:

1. ADA 2010: American Diabetes Association. Standards of medical care in diabetes – 2010. Diabetes Care. 2010;33(Suppl 1):S11–S61. [http://care.diabetesjournals.org/content/33/Supplement_1/S11]

---

[20] ADA 2009 – Although any form of insulin is effective, infusion is preferred because of short half-life and easy titration.

[21] ADA 2006/AAFP 2013 – No bolus needed if given at this rate.

[22] ADA 2009/AAFP 2013 – Done cautiously because of risk of cerebral edema.

[23] AAFP 2013 – No particular recommendation for either potassium phosphate, potassium acetate, or potassium chloride.

[24] AAFP 2013 recommends ≥6.9.

[25] ADA 2009 – There are no studies on phosphate repletion in HHS.

[26] ADA 2009 – No recommendations for Mg.

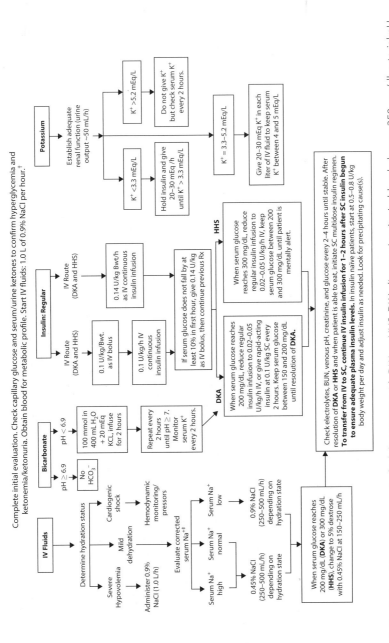

FIGURE 9-1. Protocol for management of adult patients with DKA or HHS. DKA diagnostic criteria: blood glucose 250 mg/dl, arterial pH 7.3, bicarbonate 15 mEq/l, and moderate ketonuria or ketonemia. HHS diagnostic criteria: serum glucose >600 mg/dl, arterial pH >7.3, serum bicarbonate >15 mEq/l, and minimal ketonuria and ketonemia.

†15–20 ml/kg/h;

‡Serum Na should be corrected for hyperglycemia (for each 100 mg/dl glucose 100 mg/dl, add 1.6 mEq to sodium value for corrected serum value).

Abbreviations: Bwt, body weight; IV, intravenous; SC, subcutaneous.

2. ADA 2016: American Diabetes Association. 13. Diabetes care in the hospital. Diabetes Care. 2016;39(Suppl 1):S99–S104. [http://care .diabetesjournals.org/content/39/Supplement_1/S99]

3. AACE/ACE 2015: Handelsman Y, Bloomgarden ZT, Grunberger G, et al. American Association of Clinical Endocrinologists and American College of Endocrinology – clinical practice guidelines for developing a diabetes mellitus comprehensive care plan – 2015. Endocr Pract. 2015;21(Suppl 1): 1–87. [https://www.aace.com/publications/guidelines]

4. ACP 2011: Qaseem A, Humphrey LL, Chou R, Clinical Guidelines Committee of the American College of Physicians. Use of intensive insulin therapy for the management of glycemic control in hospitalized patients: a clinical practice guideline from the American College of Physicians. Ann Intern Med. 2011;154(4):260–267. [http://annals.org/aim/article/746815/ use-intensive-insulin-therapy-management-glycemic-control-hospitalized-patients-clinical]

5. AACE/ADA 2009: Moghissi ES, Korytkowski MT, DiNardo M, et al. American Association of Clinical Endocrinologists and American Diabetes Association consensus statement on inpatient glycemic control. Diabetes Care. 2009;32(6):1119–1131. [https://www.aace.com/files/ inpatientglycemiccontrolconsensusstatement.pdf]

6. ADA 2013: American Diabetes Association – diagnosis and classification of diabetes Mellitus. Diabetes Care. 2013;36(Suppl 1):S67–S74. [http://care .diabetcsjournals.org/content/36/Supplement_1/S67]

7. ES 2012: Umpierrez GE, Hellman R, Korytkowski MT, et al. Management of hyperglycemia in hospitalized patients in non-critical care setting: an endocrine society clinical practice guideline. J Clin Endocrinol Metab. 2012;97(1):16–38. [https://www.guideline.gov/summaries/ summary/35255?]

8. ADA 2009: Kitabchi AE, Umpierrez GE, Miles JM, Fisher JN. Hyperglycemic crises in adult patients with diabetes. Diabetes Care. 2009;32(7):1335–1343. [http://care.diabetesjournals.org/content/32/7/1335]

9. AAFP 2013: Westerberg DP. Diabetic ketoacidosis: evaluation and treatment. Am Fam Physician. 2013;87(5):337–346. [http://www.aafp.org/ afp/2013/0301/p337.html]

Perioperative Considerations

David Araujo

ASSESSING PERIOPERATIVE CARDIOVASCULAR RISK

Initial Assessment (ACC/AHA 2014)

1. Determine timing of proposed surgery (emergency, urgent, time-sensitive, or elective – see Table 10-1) and risk of operation for major adverse cardiac event (MACE); divide risk of operation into two categories, low risk (risk of MACE <1%) or elevated risk (risk of MACE >1%); MACE is defined as death or myocardial infarction

2. Use a risk calculator to more precisely calculate surgical risk; options include the revised cardiac risk index (RCRI), Gupta perioperative cardiac risk, or American College of Surgeons NSQIP risk calculator

3. Assess patient's risk factors; for patients with valvular heart disease, obtain a preoperative echocardiogram if it has not been performed within the past 1 year or if there has been a significant change in clinical status

4. Assess functional capacity; if the patient can perform at least 4 METS of work (walk two blocks on level ground, or carry two bags of groceries up one flight of stairs, without symptoms consistent with typical angina), they can proceed to surgery without further testing, even if they have elevated risk; if unable to perform 4 METS of work, do further cardiac workup if this will impact patient/clinician decision making; if patient willing to undergo PCI or CABG, then perform pharmacologic stress testing

5. Adjunctive assessments
   a. 12 lead electrocardiogram
      i. Reasonable in patients with known heart disease, significant arrhythmia, peripheral arterial disease, cerebrovascular disease except for those undergoing low-risk surgery
      ii. Routine ECG is not useful for asymptomatic patients undergoing low-risk surgical procedures
   b. Assessment of left ventricular function
      i. Reasonable in patients with dyspnea of unknown origin or patients with known heart failure with worsening dyspnea

TABLE 10-1

DEFINITIONS OF URGENCY AND RISK (ADAPTED FROM ACC/AHA 2014)	
Timing of Procedure	**Level of Risk**
Emergency	Life or limb threatening if no operation, no or very limited time for clinical evaluation, operation must be performed in <6 hours
Urgent	Life or limb threatening if no operation within 6–24 hours, may be time for limited clinical evaluation
Time sensitive	A delay of >1–6 weeks to allow for clinical evaluation will negatively affect outcome
Elective	Procedure could be delayed for up to 1 year

    c. Exercise testing
        i. Reasonable to forgo exercise testing and cardiac imaging in a patient with elevated risk but excellent functional capacity, >10 METS
        ii. For those patients with functional capacity >4 METS–10 METS, it is reasonable to forgo exercise testing and cardiac imaging
        iii. If <4 METS or unknown functional capacity, it is reasonable to perform exercise testing with cardiac imaging if it will change perioperative management

Medical Management (ACC/AHA 2014)

1. Timing of surgery in patients with previous PCI
    a. Delay elective noncardiac surgery:
        i. 14 days after balloon angioplasty
        ii. 30 days after bare-metal stent placement
        iii. 365 days after drug-eluting stent placement
2. Perioperative beta blocker therapy
    a. Continue beta blockers for those patients who have been taking them chronically prior to surgery
    b. Do not initiate beta blockers on the day of surgery
    c. Consider starting beta blockers at least 2 days prior to surgery in patients with intermediate or high risk of myocardial ischemia noted on preoperative evaluation, or three or more risk factors (diabetes, heart failure, CAD, renal insufficiency, cerebrovascular disease)
3. Perioperative statin therapy
    a. Continue statins in patients who have been taking them chronically
    b. Consider initiating statins for patient undergoing vascular surgery
4. Perioperative alpha-2 agonists
    a. Do not use for prevention of cardiac events in patients undergoing noncardiac surgery

5. Perioperative angiotensin-converting enzyme inhibitors
   a. It is reasonable to continue angiotensin-converting enzyme inhibitors or angiotensin receptor blockers if the patient is taking them chronically
6. Perioperative antiplatelet agents
   a. Reasonable to continue aspirin in patients undergoing nonemergency/nonurgent noncardiac surgery who have not had coronary stenting
   b. Continue dual antiplatelet therapy (DAPT) in the patient undergoing urgent noncardiac surgery in the first 4–6 weeks after bare-metal stent or drug-eluting stent placement unless the relative risk of bleeding outweighs the benefit of prevention of stent thrombosis

Source:

1. ACC/AHA 2014: Fleisher LA, Fleischmann KE, Auerbach AD, et al. 2014 ACC/AHA guideline on perioperative cardiovascular evaluation and management of patients undergoing non-cardiac surgery: executive summary: a report of the American College of Cardiology/American Heart Association Task Force on Practice Guidelines. Circulation. 2014;130:2215–2245. [https://www.ncbi.nlm.nih.gov/pubmed/25085962]

PERIOPERATIVE ANTICOAGULATION

Initial Assessment

1. Determine type of operative procedure and its relative risk for perioperative bleeding and the type of anticoagulation agent being used, i.e., vitamin K antagonist (VKA); antiplatelet therapy (aspirin (ASA)), clopidogrel, prasugrel; non-vitamin K antagonist oral anticoagulant (NOAC) including dabigatran, rivaroxaban, apixaban, and edoxaban; perioperative bridging with either heparin (unfractionated heparin (UFH)) or enoxaparin (LMWH)
   a. Risk factor screening (STS 2012)
      i. Patients with advanced age, diminished red blood cell volume, complex operations, heart valve operations, thoracic aortic vascular procedure, urgent operations, chronic conditions such as renal failure, represent a subset at greater risk for perioperative bleeding
   b. Laboratory testing (AHA 2017)
      i. Perform prior to any procedure, if indicated by agent
         1. Measure prothrombin time (PT) for any patient on VKAs
         2. Measure partial thromboplastin time (PTT) for patients on UFH
         3. Do not routinely test, but a normal PTT and thrombin time most likely excludes therapeutic levels of dabigatran
         4. Undetectable anti-Xa activity level likely excludes clinical levels of rivaroxaban, apixaban, and edoxaban

Management of Specific Clinical Situations

1. VKA (ACCP 2012)
   a. Minor dermatologic, dental, and ophthalmologic procedures do not require interruption of VKA; optimize local hemostatic measures in these patients
   b. For those patients who require temporary interruption of VKA:
      i. Stop 5 days before the procedure
      ii. Resume 12–24 hours after the procedure
   c. Bridging anticoagulation is suggested for those patients with a mechanical heart valve, atrial fibrillation, or venous thromboembolism (VTE) at high risk for thromboembolism during interruption of VKA therapy; consider patient preference as to the relative value placed on avoiding preoperative bleeding versus the risk of thromboembolism; if bridging anticoagulation with IV UFH, discontinue UFH 4–6 hours prior to surgery; if bridging anticoagulation with low-molecular-weight heparin (LMWH) give the last dose 24 hours prior to surgery
   d. Resume LMWH in patients undergoing high-bleeding risk surgery in 48–72 hours after surgery, and in patients undergoing non-high-bleeding risk surgery in 24 hours after surgery
2. Antiplatelet medications (ASA, clopidogrel, prasugrel) (ACCP 2012)
   a. Do not stop ASA or clopidogrel for minor dermatologic, dental, or ophthalmologic procedures
   b. Noncardiac surgery
      i. Continue ASA in those patients at high or moderate risk for cardiovascular events
      ii. Stop ASA 7–10 days prior to procedure for those patients at low risk for cardiovascular events
   c. Coronary artery bypass surgery (CABG)
      i. Continue ASA
      ii. Stop clopidogrel/prasugrel 5 days before surgery; if on DAPT, continue the ASA
   d. Patients with coronary stents on DAPT:
      i. Defer surgery for 6 weeks after placement of a bare-metal stent
      ii. Defer surgery for 6 months after placement of a drug-eluting stent
      iii. If surgery is required for these patients, continue DAPT around the time of surgery
3. NOACs (dabigatran, rivaroxaban, apixaban, and edoxaban) (AHA 2017)
   a. Minor dental, dermatologic, ophthalmologic, or endoscopic without biopsy procedures do not require cessation of NOACs
   b. Moderate-high bleeding risk procedures – Stop NOACs based on the elimination half-life; for apixaban, rivaroxaban, and edoxaban stop 24 hours prior to procedure; for dabigatran, stop 24 hours prior to the

procedure for CrCl >80 mL/min, 36 hours for CrCl 50–79 mL/min, and 48 hours before for CrCl <50 mL/min

c. Do not use bridging therapy with UFH or LMWH for patients on chronic NOAC therapy

d. Reversal of dabigatran if needed prior to surgery is with idarucizumab given as two consecutive IV infusions of 2.5 g each; prothrombin complex concentrates (PCC) may also be given for dabigatran, apixaban, rivaroxaban, and edoxaban if needed prior to surgery

Sources:

1. STS 2012: Ferraris VA, Saha SP, Oestreich JH, et al. 2012 update to the Society of Thoracic Surgeons guideline on use of antiplatelet drugs in patients having cardiac and noncardiac operations. Ann Thorac Surg. 2012 Nov;94(5):1761–1781. [https://www.ncbi.nlm.nih.gov/pubmed/23098967]

2. AHA 2017: Raval AN, Cigarroa JE, Chung MK, et al. Management of patients on non-vitamin antagonist oral anticoagulants in the acute care and periprocedural setting: a scientific statement from the American Heart Association. Circulation. 2017;135(10):e604–e633. [https://www.ncbi.nlm.nih.gov/pubmed/28167634]

3. ACCP 2012: Douketis JD, Spyropoulos AC, Spencer FA, et al. Perioperative management of antithrombotic therapy: antithrombotic therapy and prevention of thrombosis, 9th ed: American College of Chest Physicians evidence-based clinical practice guidelines. Chest. 2012;141(2 Suppl):e326S–e350S. https://www.ncbi.nlm.nih.gov/pubmed/22315266]

ANTIMICROBIAL PROPHYLAXIS FOR SURGERY

Initial Assessment (IDSA/ASHP 2013)

1. Assess type of procedure, patient allergies, and antimicrobial agents available

2. For most procedures, cefazolin is the drug of choice; for patients with known methicillin-resistant *Staphylococcus aureus* (MRSA) colonization or previous MRSA surgical site infections (SSI), vancomycin can be used

3. Use SSI surveillance data to guide antimicrobial agent choice

4. Administer antimicrobial prophylaxis 60 minutes prior to incision; for those agents with a prolonged administration time, such as vancomycin or fluoroquinolones, administer 120 minutes prior to incision; optimum duration of antimicrobials is one dose; for longer procedures, re-dose if the procedure duration exceeds two half-lives of the drug or if there is excessive blood loss; there is no evidence to support continuing antibiotics until drains are removed

5. Determine *S. aureus* nasal colonization and use of mupirocin ointment intranasally if colonized for cardiac procedures, spinal procedures,

hip and other orthopedic procedures where there is implantation; the optimum time for decontamination with mupirocin is 5 days prior to the procedure

Management of Specific Clinical Situations (IDSA/ASHP 2013)

1. Cardiac procedures
   a. Give cefazolin single dose
   b. Give clindamycin or vancomycin if beta lactam allergy
   c. Give mupirocin intranasally for patient with documented *S. aureus* colonization
2. Cardiac device insertion procedures
   a. Give cefazolin single dose
   b. Give clindamycin or vancomycin for beta lactam allergy
3. Thoracic procedures
   a. Give cefazolin single dose
   b. Give clindamycin or vancomycin for beta lactam allergy
4. Gastrointestinal procedures
   a. Give cefazolin single dose
   b. Give clindamycin or vancomycin plus gentamicin, or aztreonam, or fluoroquinolone for beta lactam allergy for any procedures in which the lumen of the intestinal tract is entered
5. Biliary tract procedures
   a. Cefazolin single dose
   b. Give clindamycin, or vancomycin plus gentamicin, or aztreonam, or fluoroquinolone; or metronidazole plus gentamicin for open biliary procedures
   c. Alternative regimens include ampicillin-sulbactam, or cefotetan, cefoxitin, ceftriaxone
   d. No antibiotic prophylaxis in low-risk patients undergoing elective laparoscopic cholecystectomies; high-risk patients (age >70 years, diabetes, open cholecystectomy, acute cholecystitis, jaundice, pregnancy, immunosuppression) require antimicrobial prophylaxis
6. Appendectomy
   a. Give single dose of cephalosporin with anaerobic activity (cefoxitin or cefotetan), or cefazolin plus metronidazole
   b. Give clindamycin plus gentamicin, or aztreonam, or a fluoroquinolone and metronidazole plus gentamicin in beta lactam allergy
7. Hernia repair procedures
   a. Give cefazolin single dose
   b. Give clindamycin or vancomycin for beta lactam allergy
8. Colorectal procedures
   a. Give single dose of cephalosporin with anaerobic activity (cefoxitin or cefotetan) or cefazolin plus metronidazole

b. In addition to IV prophylaxis, for most patients, oral neomycin sulfate plus oral erythromycin base or oral neomycin sulfate plus oral metronidazole given as three doses over 10 hours after mechanical bowel preparation

9. Head and neck procedures
   a. No antimicrobial prophylaxis unless there is placement of prosthetic material, then give cefazolin single dose
   b. Give clindamycin for beta lactam allergy
   c. For clean-contaminated procedures where there is increased risk of Gram-negative contamination, give clindamycin plus gentamicin

10. Neurosurgical procedures
    a. Give cefazolin single dose
    b. Give clindamycin or vancomycin for beta lactam allergy

11. Cesarean delivery
    a. Give cefazolin single dose
    b. Give clindamycin plus gentamicin for beta lactam allergy

12. Hysterectomy procedures
    a. Give cefazolin single dose
    b. Give clindamycin or vancomycin plus an aminoglycoside, aztreonam or a fluoroquinolone and metronidazole plus an aminoglycoside for beta lactam allergy

13. Orthopedic procedures
    a. No antimicrobial prophylaxis for procedures without instrumentation or implantation

14. Spinal procedures
    a. Give cefazolin single dose
    b. Give clindamycin or vancomycin for beta lactam allergy
    c. Give mupirocin intranasally for patients colonized with *S. aureus*

15. Hip fracture repair/total joint replacement
    a. Give cefazolin single dose
    b. Give clindamycin or vancomycin for beta lactam allergy
    c. Give mupirocin intranasally for patients colonized with *S. aureus*

16. Urologic procedures
    a. No antimicrobial prophylaxis for clean urologic procedures without risk factors
    b. Treat patients with preoperative urinary tract infections before the procedure
    c. For patients undergoing lower urinary tract instrumentation use a fluoroquinolone or trimethoprim-sulfamethoxazole, or cefazolin
    d. For patients with procedures entering the urinary tract, cefazolin, or fluoroquinolone, or the combination of an aminoglycoside plus metronidazole

17. Vascular procedures
    a. Give cefazolin single dose
    b. Give clindamycin or vancomycin for beta lactam allergy

Source:

1. IDSA/ASHP 2013: Bratzler DW, Dellinger ET, Olsen KM, et al. Clinical practice guidelines for antimicrobial prophylaxis in surgery. Am J Health Syst Pharm. 2013;70(3):195–283. [https://www.ncbi.nlm.nih.gov/pubmed/23461695]

Prevention of Complications

Jacob A. David
Kristi M. Schoeld

VENOUS THROMBOEMBOLISM PROPHYLAXIS

Best Practices for Prevention (ACCP 2012, ISCI 2012, NICE 2015)

1. Give low-molecular-weight heparin, unfractionated heparin, or fondaparinux to acutely ill patients at increased risk[1] of DVT
2. Use mechanical thromboprophylaxis (intermittent pneumatic compression or graded compression stockings) if at high risk for major bleeding[2]
3. Do not use any prophylaxis for acutely ill patients at low risk of VTE

Sources:

1. ACCP 2012: Kahn SR, Lim W, Dunn A, et al. Prevention of VTE in nonsurgical patients: antithrombotic therapy and prevention of thrombosis, 9th ed: American College of Chest Physicians evidence-based clinical practice guidelines. Chest. 2012;141:e195S–e226S. [https://guidelines.gov/summaries/summary/35263]
2. ISCI 2012: Kalliainen JS, Adebayo L, Agarwal Z, et al. Institute for Clinical Systems Improvement. Venous thromboembolism prophylaxis. 2012. [https://www.qualitymeasures.ahrq.gov/summaries/summary/39365]
3. NICE 2015: Venous thromboembolism: reducing the risk for patients in hospital. National Institute for Health and Care Excellence. 2015. [https://www.nice.org.uk/Guidance/CG92]
4. J Thromb Haemost 2010: Barbar S, Noventa F, Rossetto V, et al. A risk assessment model for the identification of hospitalized patients at risk for

---

[1] A Padua prediction score ≥4 suggests a patient at high risk who could benefit from prophylaxis. The score assigns 3 points each for active cancer, previous DVT, reduced mobility, known thrombophilic condition; 2 points for trauma and/or surgery in the past month; and 1 point each for age ≥70 years, heart and/or respiratory failure, acute MI or ischemic stroke, acute infection and/or rheumatologic disorder, BMI ≥30, and ongoing hormonal treatment (J Thromb Haemost. 2010).

[2] Significant risk factors for major bleeding include active gastroduodenal ulcer, bleeding actively or in the 3 months prior to admission, thrombocytopenia, elderly age, liver failure with elevated INR, renal insufficiency, acute stroke, uncontrolled systolic hypertension.

venous thromboembolism: the Padua prediction score. J Thromb Haemost. 2010;8:2450–2457. [https://www.ncbi.nlm.nih.gov/pubmed/20738765]

PRESSURE ULCERS

Best Practices for Prevention (ACP 2015, NICE 2015)

1. Perform a risk assessment on every patient
2. Use advanced static foam mattresses or overlays in patients at increased risk for pressure ulcers
3. Do not use alternating air mattresses; they do not work better than static mattresses but cost more
4. Turn high-risk patients frequently, at least every 6 hours

Sources:

1. ACP 2015: Qaseem A, Mir T, Starkey M, Denberg T. Risk assessment and prevention of pressure ulcers: a clinical practice guideline from the American College of Physicians. Ann Internal Med. 2015;162:359–369. [https://www.guideline.gov/summaries/summary/49050]
2. NICE 2015: Pressure ulcers: prevention and management. National Institute for Health and Care Excellence. 2014. [nice.org.uk/guidance/cg179]

CATHETER-RELATED BLOODSTREAM INFECTIONS

Best Practices for Prevention (IDSA/CDC 2011)

1. Use a subclavian vein[3] rather than jugular or femoral for nontunneled central venous access
2. Promptly remove any catheter that is not essential; replace catheters placed under questionable aseptic technique within 48 hours
3. Place catheters using maximal sterile technique including full barrier precautions and chlorhexidine skin prep, allowed to dry completely
4. Dress catheters with sterile dressing; consider chlorhexidine-impregnated sponge; replace on schedule, or if it becomes loose or soiled

Sources:

1. IDSA/CDC 2011: O'Grady NP, Alexander M, Burns LA, et al. Guidelines for the prevention of intravascular catheter-related infections. Clin Infect Dis. 2011;52:e1–e32. [https://www.ncbi.nlm.nih.gov/pmc/articles/PMC3106269/]
2. Crit Care Med 2011: Fragou M, Gravvanis A, Dimitriou V, et al. Real-time ultrasound-guided subclavian vein cannulation versus the landmark

[3]For central venous catheters, use of real-time ultrasound guidance may reduce complications and facilitate placement in patients for whom a landmark-based approach is difficult (Crit Care Med. 2011).

method in critical care patients: a prospective randomized study. Crit Care Med. 2011;39:1607–1612. [https://www.ncbi.nlm.nih.gov/pubmed/21494105]

CATHETER-RELATED URINARY TRACT INFECTIONS

Best Practices for Prevention (IDSA 2010)

1. Place indwelling catheters only when necessary; a trained professional should insert using sterile technique; institutions should have criteria for appropriate indications and require a physician order for placement
2. Remove indwelling catheters as soon as possible; institutions should have nursing-driven or EHR-driven removal protocols
3. Use intermittent catheterization when appropriate as an alternative to an indwelling catheter because it carries a lower risk of catheter-associated bacteriuria
4. Use a closed catheter system when an indwelling catheter as necessary, keep the drainage bag below the level of the patient's bladder, and consider a catheter coated with antimicrobials
5. Do not use systemic antibiotic prophylaxis, methamphetamine salts, cranberry products, catheter irrigation, or antibiotics in the drainage bag to prevent catheter-associated UTI

Source:

1. IDSA 2010: Hooton TM, Bradley SF, Cardenas DD, et al. Diagnosis, prevention, and treatment of catheter-associated urinary tract infection in adults: 2009 international clinical practice guidelines from the Infectious Diseases Society of America. Clin Infect Dis. 2010;50:625–663. [https://www.ncbi.nlm.nih.gov/pubmed/20175247]

ACUTE KIDNEY INJURY

Assessing Risk

1. Identifying acute kidney injury (AKI) in patients with acute illness (NICE 2013)
   a. Investigate for AKI, by measuring serum Cr and comparing with baseline, in adults with acute illness if any of the following are present:
      i. CKD (adults with eGFR <60 mL/min/m^2)
      ii. Heart failure
      iii. Liver disease
      iv. Diabetes
      v. History of AKI
      vi. Oliguria (urine output <0.5 mL/kg/h)

       vii. Neurologic or cognitive impairment or disability

      viii. Hypovolemia

       ix. Use of nephrotoxic drugs in the past week, including iodinated contrast

       x. Symptoms or history of urologic obstruction

       xi. Sepsis

      xii. Age >65 years

2. Identifying AKI in patients with no obvious acute illness (NICE 2013)

   a. In patients with CKD, a rise in serum Cr may indicate AKI rather than a worsening or their CKD; consider AKI with any of the following:

       i. CKD stage 3B, 4, or 5, or urologic disease

      ii. New onset or significant worsening of urologic symptoms

     iii. Symptoms or signs of multi-organ disease including the kidneys

3. Assessing risk factors in adults having surgery (NICE 2013)

   a. Increased risk is associated with:

       i. Emergency surgery, especially in the setting of sepsis or hypovolemia

      ii. Intraperitoneal surgery

     iii. CKD (eGFR <60 mL/min/m^2)

      iv. Diabetes

       v. Heart failure

      vi. Age ≥65 years

      vii. Liver disease

     viii. Use of nephrotoxic drugs in the perioperative period

4. Assessing risk factors in adults having iodinated contrast agents (NICE 2013, KDIGO 2012)

   a. Before nonemergent imaging, check for CKD by measuring eGFR or checking for a result within the past 3 months

   b. Before emergent or nonemergent imaging, assess for risk of AKI; include the risk of developing AKI in informed consent discussions for the procedure

   c. Consider alternative imaging in patients at increased risk; increased risk is associated with:

       i. CKD (eGFR <40 mL/min/m^2)

      ii. Diabetes with CKD

     iii. Heart failure

      iv. Renal transplant

       v. Age ≥75 years

      vi. Hypovolemia

     vii. Larger volumes of contrast agents

    viii. Intra-arterial administration of contrast

Prevention

1. Assess hospitalized patients to recognize and respond to oliguria[4] (NICE 2013, KDIGO 2012)

   a. Discuss care with pharmacist to optimize medications and dosing in patients with or at risk for AKI

   b. Consider holding ACEi and ARBs in adults with diarrhea, vomiting, or sepsis

   c. Monitor serum Cr regularly in patients with or at risk for AKI

   d. In the absence of shock, use isotonic crystalloids (IVF) rather than colloids as initial management for volume expansion in patients with or at risk for AKI

   e. In patients with vasomotor shock, use vasopressors in conjunction with IVF in patients with or at risk for AKI

   f. Do not use diuretics to prevent or treat AKI except in the setting of volume overload

   g. Do not use low-dose dopamine to prevent or treat AKI

   h. Do not use fenoldopam to prevent or treat AKI

   i. Do not use atrial natriuretic peptide (ANP) to prevent or treat AKI

   j. Do not use recombinant human insulin-like growth factor 1 to prevent or treat AKI

2. Prevent contrast-induced AKI (CI-AKI) (NICE 2013, KDIGO 2012)

   a. Give IVF (isotonic sodium bicarb or 0.9% sodium chloride) to adults having iodinated contrast if they are at increased risk of AKI due to contrast OR they have an acute illness; do not use oral fluids alone

   b. Use the lowest possible dose of contrast media in patients at risk for CI-AKI

   c. Use either iso-osmolar or low-osmolar iodinated contrast media, rather than high-osmolar contrast media, in patients at risk for CI-AKI

   d. Consider holding ACEi and ARBs in adults have a contrast study if they have CKD with eGFR <40

   e. Discuss care with nephrology before giving contrast to adults with contraindications to IVF if they are at risk for CI-AKI or have an acute illness or are on dialysis

   f. Use oral NAC together with IV isotonic crystalloids in patients at increased risk for CI-AKI

   g. Do not use theophylline to prevent CI-AKI

   h. Do not use fenoldopam to prevent CI-AKI

   i. Do not use prophylactic intermittent hemodialysis (IHD) or hemofiltration (HF) for contrast-media removal in patients at risk for CI-AKI

[4]Oliguria: urine output <0.5 mL/kg/h

3. Prevent aminoglycoside-related AKI (KDIGO 2012)
   a. Do not use aminoglycosides for the treatment of infection unless no suitable less nephrotoxic alternative is available
   b. In patients with normal renal function, give aminoglycosides as a single daily dose rather than multiple daily doses
   c. If using multiple daily dosing of aminoglycoside for more than 24 hours, monitor aminoglycoside levels
   d. If using single daily dosing of aminoglycoside for more than 48 hours, monitor aminoglycoside levels
   e. Use topical or local applications of aminoglycosides rather than IV when feasible
4. Prevent amphotericin B-related AKI (KDIGO 2012)
   a. Use lipid formations of amphotericin B rather than conventional formulations
   b. Use azole antifungal agents and/or the echinocandins rather than conventional amphotericin B if equal therapeutic efficacy
5. Prevent AKI in the critically ill (KDIGO 2012)
   a. Do not use NAC (N-acetylcysteine) to prevent AKI in critically ill patients with hypotension
   b. Do not use oral or IV NAC to prevent postsurgical AKI
      i. Do not select off-pump coronary artery bypass graft surgery solely to reduce perioperative AKI or need for dialysis
      ii. Use insulin therapy targeting plasma glucose 110–149
      iii. Provide nutrition preferentially via the enteral route
      iv. Achieve a total energy intake of 20–30 kcal/kg/day in patients with any stage of AKI
      v. Avoid restriction of protein intake for the aim of avoiding dialysis
         1. Administer 0.8–1.0 g/kg/day of protein in patients with AKI not on dialysis
         2. Administer 1.0–1.5 g/kg/day of protein in patients with AKI on dialysis

Sources:

1. NICE 2013: National Clinical Guideline Centre. Acute kidney injury. Prevention, detection and management of acute kidney injury up to the point of renal replacement therapy. London (UK): National Institute for Health and Care Excellence (NICE);2013 Aug. 39 p. (clinical guideline; no. 169). [https://www.nice.org.uk/guidance/CG169]
2. KDIGO 2012: KDIGO clinical practice guideline for acute kidney injury. Kidney Int Suppl. 2012 Mar;2(1):1–138. [http://www.guideline.gov/summaries/summary/38024]

CHOOSING WISELY – SOCIETY OF HOSPITAL MEDICINE

Prevent Catheter-Associated Urinary Tract Infections

1. Avoid catheters for incontinence, convenience, and output monitoring
2. Only use urinary catheters in critical illness, urinary obstruction, hospice care, or for up to 48 hours after a urologic procedure
3. Weigh patients to monitor diuresis

Give Acid-Reducing Medications to Treat Disease, Not to Prevent Stress Ulcers

1. Medication for stress ulcer prophylaxis carries more risk (pneumonia, *Clostridium difficile*, unnecessary cost) than benefit outside of the ICU

Transfuse Red Blood Cells to Treat Signs of Impaired Oxygen Delivery; Don't Transfuse to an Arbitrary Hemoglobin Level

1. A hemoglobin of 7–8 g/dL is usually sufficient in stable patients
2. Active coronary syndrome, heart failure, or stroke may merit a higher hemoglobin target[5]

Place a Time Limit on Use of Telemetry Outside the ICU

1. Prolonged telemetry may increase cost and generate false positives
2. Develop hospital protocols with reference to published guidelines (i.e., in patients with low risk of a cardiac cause of chest pain, telemetry is of little measurable benefit)

Draw Labs When They're Necessary, and Don't When They're Not

1. Daily blood counts and chemistries are often unnecessary
2. The aggregate effect of phlebotomy can result in clinically significant blood loss

Source:

1. Society of Hospital Medicine: Choosing wisely. Philadelphia (PA);2013. [http://www.choosingwisely.org/societies/society-of-hospital-medicine-adult/]

---

[5]See page 151 for specific recommendations.

End-of-Life Care

Leslie-Lynn Pawson
Heather Nennig

THE PALLIATIVE CARE INTERVENTION

Initial Assessment

1. Recognize when a person may be in the last days of life (PCNOW #3)
   a. "Actively dying" or "imminent death" – Progress through stages from <24 hours to 14 days depending on prior health of patient
      i. Early: Bed bound, loss of interest or inability to eat, increased sleep/delirium
      ii. Middle: Further mental decline to obtundation
      iii. Late: Death "rattle," coma, fever, fluctuating respirations, mottled extremities
      iv. Actively dying: Physical changes include decreased BP; fluctuating HR, temperature, and respirations; clamminess; skin changes (flushed, bluish, pale yellowish pallor); congestion; extremities cool and purplish/blotchy; coma prior to death (NICE 2015)
2. Gather information (NICE 2015)
   a. Patient's physiological, psychological, social, and spiritual needs
   b. Current signs and symptoms (including symptoms of imminent death listed above)
   c. PMH, clinical context, and underlying diagnosis
   d. Patient's goals, wishes, and views about future care
3. Use a multidisciplinary team and consult if any uncertainty whether patient is declining, stabilizing, or recovering (NICE 2015)
4. Monitor for changes every 24 hours (NICE 2015)

Communicate Prognosis to Patient, Surrogate Decision Makers, and Family

1. Determine the needs and expectations of those dying (NICE 2015)
   a. If another person is desired to be present for decision making
   b. Current level of understanding of patient about his/her dying

    c. Cognitive status or any communicative special need

    d. Level of detail about prognosis

    e. Other cultural, religious, social, or spiritual needs

2. Identify most appropriate team member to explain prognosis (NICE 2015)

3. Discuss and document prognosis and preferences (NICE 2015)

    a. Give accurate information, explain uncertain, avoid false "hope"

    b. Discuss fears and anxieties

    c. Contact information for care team/family

    d. Preferences (if any) for last days of life

4. Anticipate common questions from family (PCNOW #29)

    a. "Is he in pain; how do we know?"

    b. "Aren't we just starving him to death?"

    c. "Should I/we stay by the bedside?"

    d. "Can he hear what we are saying?"

    e. "What do we do after death?"

5. Share decision making in advanced care planning (NICE 2015)

    a. Determine patient's mental capacity/level of involvement in decision making

    b. Determine if patient has an advance directive, durable power of attorney (DPOA)

    c. Determine patient's current goals/wishes or any cultural, religious, social, or spiritual preferences

    d. Offer provider contact details including afterhours contact information

    e. Provide individualized care

        i. Establish early resources (e.g., meals, equipment, caretaker support)

        ii. Determine goals/wishes, preferred care setting, symptom management, care for after death, resource needs

        iii. Record in chart and discuss with patient

        iv. Revisit frequently the care plan with patient and family and update as needed

        v. If unable to meet wishes of patient, explain why

        vi. Consult specialist advice if additional support needed (e.g., palliative care team)

Acute Medical Management

1. Wean medications when impending death is recognized; taper certain medications to avoid withdrawal symptoms (i.e., proton pump inhibitors, steroids, chronic benzodiazepines, antidepressants)

2. Assess and manage hydration (PCNOW #133, # 220, # 134, # 313, NICE 2015)

    a. Oral hydration

        i. Support the dying person to drink if they wish to

      ii. Provide oral care by brushing teeth gently or wiping oral surfaces with water moistened swab

  b. Non-oral hydration (if desired by patient and family)

      i. Review the arguments for and against non-oral hydration; non-oral hydration is considered a medical intervention, not ordinary care; as such, there is no legal or ethical imperative to provide it unless the benefits outweigh the burdens

      ii. Do not place enteral tubes solely for hydration management in the last few days or weeks of life; provide other less burdensome methods of hydration

      iii. Use IV hydration in the short term only as a time-limited trial to see if it relieves suffering

      iv. Consider hypodermoclysis (subcutaneous infusion) if IV site becomes a problem and/or patient desires freedom from IV poles and pumps; use infusion sets with 25- to 27-gauge needles and infuse 0.9% sodium chloride or 5% dextrose and ½ normal saline at 70–100 mL/h continuous infusion or 500 mL bolus over 1 hour BID; the upper chest is the site most commonly used

3. Assess and manage physical pain and pain medication side effects (PCNOW #20, #54, #92, #28, NICE 2015)

  a. Assess dying person's level and type of pain using 0–10 scale or FACES scale or mild/moderate/severe descriptor

  b. Assess type and cause of pain and treat cause when possible (e.g., abdominal pain from constipation or urinary retention)

  c. Match the medicine for pain to the severity of pain and use dying patient's preference for how pain medication is administered

  d. If using an opioid infusion in the dying patient (PCNOW #54)

      i. If patient is already on opioids for pain, calculate an equianalgesic dose of currently used opioids; then convert this to an equianalgesic basal rate; example: a patient on oral extended release morphine 60 mg q12, now unable to swallow; 60 mg q 12 = 120 mg/24 hours PO morphine = 40 mg IV morphine/24 hours = approximately 2 mg/h IV infusion basal rate

      ii. If the patient is opioid naïve, give a loading dose when starting the infusion; e.g., for a 1 mg/h basal rate, give 2–5 mg loading dose

      iii. Choose a bolus dose for breakthrough pain; a bolus dose of 50%–150% of the hourly rate is a place to start; e.g., for a morphine infusion of 2 mg/h, choose a starting bolus dose of 1–3 mg

      iv. Dose at an interval of q10–20 minutes because the peak analgesic effect from an IV bolus dose is 10–20 minutes

v. Adjust bolus dose size every 30–60 minutes until control of pain is achieved without unacceptable toxicities

vi. Reassess basal dose no more frequently than q8 hours using number of bolus doses that were necessary

vii. Do not increase the basal rate by more than 100% at any one time

viii. When patients become anuric close to death, continuous dosing may be discontinued in favor of bolus dosing to prevent metabolite accumulation and agitated delirium

e. Manage breathlessness and medication side effects (PCNOW #27, NICE 2015)

i. Identify and treat reversible causes of breathlessness in the dying patient (e.g., manage malignant pleural effusion with surgically placed pleural drainage catheter); use when the patient is in the dying trajectory; allow their identified goals of care to guide the extent of workup for reversible causes

ii. Do not start oxygen to manage breathlessness; use only in known symptomatic hypoxemia; do not base on pulse oximetry; deliver by nasal cannula preferably not by mask; dyspnea does not correlate with O_2 saturation or respiratory rate

iii. Use sitting up leaning, forward positioning, fan, open window; line of sight to open space

iv. Use opioids for end-of-life dyspnea

1. If the patient is opioid naïve, 5–10 mg oral morphine or 2–4 mg parenteral morphine

2. If dyspnea is acute and severe, 1–3 mg IV q 1–2 hours

3. Can be more aggressive if needed (e.g., continuous IV infusion)

4. Use higher doses if on chronic opioids

5. Use anxiolytics to relieve anxiety associated with breathlessness (i.e., lorazepam 0.5–1 mg PO/SL/SC/IV q2 hours)

f. Manage nausea, vomiting, and medication side effects (PCNOW #5, #25, NICE 2015, Cancer Care Ontario)

i. Assess for likely causes in the dying patient; VOMIT acronym (Vestibular/Obstruction/Metabolic/Inflammation/Toxin) can help

ii. When considering medicines to manage nausea in the dying patient, consider the drug based receptor implicated in cause

1. If cause is opioid use, consider decreasing dose of opioid or switching opioids

2. If cause is opioids and decide to use medications, use dopamine antagonists (e.g., prochlorperazine 10–20 mg PO q6 hour or 25 mg PR q6–12 hour OR haloperidol 0.5–2 mg PO/SC/IV q4–6 hour OR metoclopramide 10–20 mg PO/SC/IV q4–6 hours)

3. If cause is obstructive bowel disorders in the dying patient, use octreotide 100–400 mcg SC/IV q8 hour (NICE 2015)

g. Manage terminal delirium: Hypoactive and hyperactive/agitation (PCNOW #1, #60, NICE 2015, Cancer Care Ontario)

    i. Recognize terminal (nonreversible) delirium; this is delirium in a patient in the final days/weeks of life, where treatment of the underlying cause is impossible, impractical, or not consistent with the goals of care

    ii. Assess for associated treatable cause. Examples include unrelieved pain, full bladder, full rectum, hyponatremia, hypoxemia, medications such as anticholinergics (e.g., anti-secretion drugs, antiemetics, antihistamines, tricyclic antidepressants, etc.), sedative-hypnotics (e.g., benzodiazepines), and opioids; decrease doses, discontinue/wean medication, and rotate/change opioid when possible

    iii. Use non-pharmacological interventions first

        1. Limit the sensory stimulation in the environment as needed by using soft lighting and gentle handling

        2. Increase sensory input as needed by providing hearing aids, glasses, calendar, and clock; ask relatives/friends to stay by the patient; frequent reminders of time/place, well-lit daytime, dim nightlight

        3. Pharmacological interventions

            a. Antipsychotics/neuroleptics drug of choice

                i. Haloperidol is administered in a dose-escalation process; start haloperidol 0.5–2 mg PO or IV or SC q1 hour PRN

                ii. If anxiety is a prominent part of a patient's delirium, a benzodiazepine may help but can cause paradoxical worsening of the delirium and agitation and should generally be avoided; lorazepam start 0.5–5 mg PO/SC/IV PRN q1 hour if PO, q30 minutes if SC, q10 minutes if IV

h. Manage secretions, noisy respirations, and medication side effects (PCNOW #109, NICE 2015)

    i. Death "rattle" is a good predictor of near death; establish whether the noise has an impact on the dying person or those close to them; reassure them that although the noise can be distressing it is unlikely to cause suffering

    ii. Position the patient on their side or in a semi-prone position to facilitate postural drainage

    iii. Frequent suctioning is disturbing to both the patient and the visitors

    iv. Pharmacological management

        1. Glycopyrrolate (1 mg PO, 0.2 mg SQ or IV): Does not cross blood-brain barrier and therefore does not cause sedation or delirium

2. Scopolamine hydrobromide (1.5 mg patch): 12 hours to onset, 24 hours to steady state
3. Hyoscyamine (0.125 mg PO or SL)
4. Atropine sulfate (1 gtt of 1% opthalmic solution; 0.1 mg SQ or IV)

i. Manage fever (PCNOW #256, National Consensus Project, ISCI 2013)

   i. Weigh all therapeutic options in the context of the patient's goals of care and whether a fever is distressing to the dying patient; there is no compelling reason to think that treatment of fever reduces suffering for dying, unresponsive patients

   ii. Discontinue any non-essential drugs if drug-induced fever is suspected

   iii. Use a fan

   iv. Antipyretics – The order can state "PRN for symptomatic fever" to discourage focus on the temperature measurement alone

   v. Acetaminophen 650–1000 mg PO/PR/IV q4–6 hours PRN (maximum dose 4 g/day) is considered first line given its low side-effect profile OR

   vi. NSAIDs (oral, IV, rectal, subcutaneous) are also effective; naproxen 250 mg q12 hours is particularly effective in neoplastic fever

Management After Death

1. "Symptoms" of death (PCNOW #149)
   a. No breathing or HR
   b. Bowel/bladder incontinence
   c. Non-responsive
   d. Eyelids slightly open with eyes and pupils fixed
   e. Jaw relaxed and mouth slightly open

2. Pronouncing or declaring death (PCNOW #4)
   a. Before entering the room:
      i. Ask nurse/staff whether death was expected or sudden, if any family present and if an interpreter is required.
      ii. Determine if autopsy needed/requested
      iii. Determine if organ donor network has been contacted
      iv. Briefly review medical (cause of death, length of stay) and family concerns (faith/clergy? who is family?)
   b. Pronouncement
      i. ID patient by hospital tag
      ii. Check for responsiveness but avoid painful stimuli if family present
      iii. Auscultate for (absent) heart sounds, palpate carotid pulse
      iv. Observe and auscultate for (absent) respirations

    v. Determine pupil position and (absent) light reflex

    vi. Record date and time of assessment

  c. Documentation

    i. "Called to pronounce [name]"; record physical exam

    ii. Note date and time and whether family (and attending physician) notified

    iii. Document autopsy acceptance or decline, natural death, or coroner notified

    iv. For death certificate: Cause of death, time between onset of condition and death, contribution of alcohol or tobacco

  d. Communicating with family and friends (PCNOW #4)

    i. Introduce yourself and ask each family members' name and relationship

    ii. Empathize: "I'm sorry for your loss," "This must be very difficult for you"

    iii. Explain your role (pronouncement) and if they'd like to stay

    iv. Ask if any questions, want to speak to chaplain

Sources:

1. National Consensus Project: Clinical practice guidelines for quality palliative care. National Consensus Project for Quality Palliative Care. 2nd ed;2009. [http://www.nationalcoalitionhpc.org/]

2. National Guideline Clearinghouse. Care of dying adults in the last days of life. London (UK): National Institute for Health and Care Excellence (NICE);2015 Dec 16. 26 p. (NICE guideline; no. 31). [https://www.guideline.gov/summaries/summary/49956]

3. ISCI 2013: McCusker M, Ceronsky L, Crone C, et al. Palliative care for adults. Bloomington (MN): Institute for Clinical Systems Improvement (ICSI);2013 Nov. 81 p. [https://www.guideline.gov/summaries/summary/47629]

4. PCNOW: Marks, S editor. Palliative care network of Wisconsin. Fast facts and concepts. [https://www.mypcnow.org/fast-facts]

5. Cancer Care Ontario: Cancer Care Ontario. (2013) Cancer Care Ontario symptom management guides (1.4) [mobile application software]. [https://itunes.apple.com/us/app/cancer-care-ontario-symptom-management-guides/id419371782?mt=8]

Index

Note: Page numbers followed by "f" and "t" represent figures and tables respectively.